Chinese Fitness

Chinese Fitness
A Mind/Body Approach

Qigong for Healthy & Joyful Living

By Qingshan Liu

YMAA Publication Center
Jamaica Plain, Mass. USA

YMAA Publication Center
38 Hyde Park Avenue
Jamaica Plain, Massachusetts, 02130

5

Publisher's Cataloging in Publication
(Prepared by Quality Books Inc.)

Liu, Ch'ing-shan.
  Chinese Fitness : a mind/body approach / Liu Qingshan.
  p. cm. — (Qigong health & healing)
  Includes bibliographical references and index.
  ISBN: 1-886969-37-X

    1. Ch'i kung—Therapeutic aspects.   2. Physical fitness.   I.
Title.
II. Title.

RM727.C54L58 1997   613.7'148
                            QBI97-40367

Disclaimer:
The author and publisher of this material are NOT RESPONSIBLE in any manner whatso-
ever for any injury which may occur through reading or following the instructions in
this manual.
The activities, physical or otherwise, described in this material may be too strenuous or
dangerous for some people, and the reader(s) should consult a physician before engaging
in them.

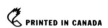 PRINTED IN CANADA

Acknowledgments

My heartfelt thanks first to my Qigong-friend of many years, Klaus Gürtner who wrote down formulations of the first draft, and improved, word for word, the subsequent changes. Sincere thanks also to Christine Behle, a participant in my course, who willingly accepted the troublesome task of typing, and produced the first clean copy of the text. For the photographs I sincerely thank Alexander Gall, Carolin Hahnemann, Claudia Zoch, and Qingmei Liu.

Further thanks to persons who read the originally corrected copy. Among these are: Professor Dr. Paul Unschuld, Chair for the History of Medicine, the University of Munich, and Dr. med. B. Ostermayr, Chief Physician of the Clinic for Natural Therapy and Internal Medicine in Munich-Harlaching.

For extensive consultations and suggestions I thank, among others, my friends: Dr. med. Herbert Hermannstaller and Dr. med. Horst Mehmel, Orthopedics, and Bernd Rossmüller physician, Anette Schrag, physician, and Rudi Pihusch, physician. For important help with the final copy I would especially like to thank Dr. Caroline Schmauser.

I would like very much to thank Professor Jackson Hershbell for the English translation of my work, and for its first correction I would like to thank Mr. Andrew Murray. Thanks to Mr. David Cole for help with the final translation, and thanks to YMAA Publication Center for making the book available in English.

Contents

B) QIGONG EXERCISE

Preface

It is very gratifying to note that in recent years Western interest in, and enjoyment of Qigong has greatly increased. This development is due to the fact that not only is Qigong easy to practice, but makes us more cheerful, and keeps us healthy. It is also suitable for all age groups, and requires no special talent or ability. Moreover, Qigong helps us to become healthy again after an illness. In China there are 100 million people practicing Qigong and it is very well known that with the help of Qigong, even severe illnesses can be successfully treated. It is no surprise that we feel balanced and relaxed after Qigong exercises.

Thanks to the tradition of my family, I became acquainted with this wonderful art when I was a child. Later, as a master of Qigong, I gave lessons, and my knowledge of Qigong deepened through my study of medicine in Beijing.

It was an interesting experience for me to realize that my students in the West could learn and do Qigong exercises as well as my students in China, if they understood the meaning and learned the essence of Qigong. It is important to understand Qigong's specific mode of action, and to recognize its differences from gymnastics and other kinds of sport. This book is intended to help people in the West to learn about Qigong from all sides, and to practice it correctly.

The exercises presented in this book are very easy to learn, and very effective. For a better overview of the illustrations, I have developed a new presentation. With the help of these illustrations you can, given their serial presentation, imitate exercises with correct breathing, and within the exact time period. There is, moreover, an accompanying videocassette available from YMAA Publication Center.

I wish you, by means of my book, joy in this ancient path to harmony of body and spirit. This book is appropriate for both beginners and advanced students, and serves as an accompanying text for my course.

Best wishes for your health, and a happy, long life.

Qingshan Liu
Munich, April 1997

CHAPTER 1

Qi and Qigong
An Introduction

◆ Traditional Chinese Medicine (TCM) and Western Medicine:

Qigong (pronounced "Chee Gong"), a method for cultivating health, originates in China, and is based on ancient knowledge. In order to understand Qigong, we will begin by comparing Traditional Chinese Medicine (TCM) with Western medicine.

Western medicine is based on natural scientific observations. It draws on the results of biological research in order to determine how organisms came about, what forms they take, and how they regulate their life functions. In anatomy, Western medicine dissects the human body so that its structures are divided, and systematically analyzes these structures. Physiology helps to determine how these anatomical structures function, and any significance they have for life. Chemical processes are analyzed by applied chemistry, and in pathology, the processes of illness are determined by tissue and organ changes.

With the aid of all these individual sciences, Western medicine differentiates between normal and pathological biological functions. It views a disturbed function of individual organ systems as the cause of illness. With the help of different disciplines such as internal medicine and surgery, Western medicine treats illnesses by "modulating" or "pacifying" these disturbed functions, and also makes use of pharmacology, the study of remedies.

TCM is not based on this kind of anatomy or physiology, but on observation of bodily reactions and interpretation of bodily experiences. To be sure, it also knows the main organs of anatomy such as the stomach, liver, etc., but it does not deal with them on an histological or cytological level. Surgery and internal medicine are well known in Traditional Chinese Medicine; it uses them, however, with a wholly different understanding. TCM is generally not interested in chemistry, but in something that is not an element of Western medicine—Qi (Life-force, Life-power).

In brief, Qi and its movements determine life. Traditional Chinese Medicine believes that you are healthy and the immune system strong if the Qi is in harmony. "If the true Qi is in harmony, how can illness arise?" *(Huang Di Nei Jing)*. If the Qi is in disharmony, there is sickness. Qi disharmony is, thus, illness itself. This concept of illness is different from that of Western medicine.

In order to examine the Qi, Chinese doctors developed diagnostic techniques that examine the tongue (for example, its shape, color, and fur), the eyes, ears, and pulse. External appearances of the body provide a basis for determining the invisible Qi and its condition.

With the following illustration, I would like to make the differences clearer between Western medicine and TCM:

The human body can be compared to a full pot cooking on the stove. Western medicine examines, in detail, how thick the pot is, and the contents of the food in the pot. Exact inventories are made, for example, of the different vitamins and proteins, and the number of calories. If the cook adds a dash of vinegar, Western medicine knows immediately how the pH changes, and so forth.

Traditional Chinese Medicine knows that the meal cooks on the stove, and should taste good. It concentrates on the appearance and quality of the food. It watches over the color, and whether it is sticky or dry, soft or hard, hot or cold. To make these observations, there are many clues unknown to Western medicine.

Suddenly there are ants in the pot! This corresponds to illness in the human body—for example, to an infection.

Western medicine asks "How can the ants can be removed?" In order to find an answer, it must first know what kind of ant is involved: whether type A, B, or even C. For specific pathogenic agents, specific remedies are applied. Several ants must be taken from the pot in order to examine them under the microscope. That corresponds, for example, to a blood sample; hence, to laboratory investigation. Because of microbiology, Western medicine knows the appearance of all disease-causing organisms.

The laboratory discovers that these are "type A" ants. Correspondingly, with the help of biochemistry and pharmacology, it discovers what remedy (e.g. antibiotic) there is against this type. Thus, the ants in the pot are challenged, and finally destroyed. However, it is well known that pharmaceuticals and medications often have undesirable side-effects: the ants will finally be destroyed, but the meal is no longer enjoyable. Nevertheless, this is regarded as healing.

There can be further problems: If by chance the remedy against type A is favorable to type B, also present, type B can now greatly increase in number, and the disease gets worse. If the type of ant is not known, Western medicine has no idea how to combat them.

While classification of pathogenic agents is important to Western medicine, Chinese Medicine concentrates on Qi and Qi-harmony. Health is guaranteed by harmony of the Qi, which forms the unity of body, soul, and mind. Thus, Chinese Medicine does not attempt to closely examine or to categorize the ants, but to check the harmony of the whole system. In regard to this example, a Chinese physician might first ask why ants are suddenly present in the food. It suggests that Qi-harmony is disturbed because the stove does not have enough heat. Thus, the ants are able to survive while in the pot. The cause of this illness is, accordingly, not ant infiltration, but the disharmony of all factors. The temperature has sunk. For an increase in temperature, the fire must be fanned. Fire is fed by wood, extinguished by water. This fact corresponds to the theory of the five phases of transformation in Chinese philosophy and medicine (see "Introduction to the Theory of the Five Elements").

Chinese medicine knows how to tell whether too little wood is available, or whether the wood used is too damp. Thus it lays on dry wood so that the fire has more heat, and drives off the ants. Chinese Medicine has left the pot untouched, and the meal remains edible. In a figurative sense, it has only made the body functional again. Although it is not interested in what type of bacteria appears, it has healed the sickness, and certainly without side-effects. In this way, Traditional Chinese Medicine has developed thousands of methods for "making fire." It knows moreover, that so long as harmony dominates—heat in this case—the ants will not return.

Traditional Chinese Medicine wants to remove the causes for the origin of disease. Healing with the help of specific medications has, on the contrary, only removed symptoms (the ants), but not the true cause. Thus, the illness can always recur again, once the effect of the medication has ceased.

By means of this example, I want only to explain the differences between the two systems, not to evaluate them. Western medicine and Traditional Chinese Medicine are by no means opposed to one another. If, for example, "making fire" in specific cases does not work quickly enough, and the ants threaten to destroy all, they must be removed "surgically"; if the pot is one day damaged by accident, you must certainly know how to repair it. In such cases, the skills and disciplines of Western medicine are indispensable.

◆ What is Qi?

"Qi" is the transcription of a Chinese ideogram, which like most Chinese ideograms, has many meanings. Qi (氣) means "Life Force". However Qi also means "Gas", "Air", "Breath", "Odor", and much more. It is a key concept of Chinese philosophy, and designates a subtle and important substance. In Traditional Chinese Medicine "Qi" stands for physiological activity, and the functional vitality of the organism; thus, it stands for life-force and life-energy.

Why does "Qi" have so many meanings, which, at first glance, have little to do with one another? An explanation is found in the fact that all these meanings are more or less bound up with breathing. Air is gaseous. It is breathed in and out. Odor is perceptible through breathing, and through breathing you gather energy. With deep inhalation and an expanded chest, you demonstrate power. Exhaustion is shown when the breath literally leaves you, and the chest collapses.

By means of Qigong exercises you can feel how the body is filled with energy when inhaling. Thus, our ancestors saw inhaled air and its resultant energy as a unity, and designated it as "Qi." Today it is known that people breathe in air, and this inhalation influences Qi-Energy. It can be disputed whether the occurrence can be viewed in different stages. In any case, the connection between air, breathing, and life energy is easily perceivable in Qigong exercises.

◆ Experiencing Qi

Even without knowing the concept of Qi, it is likely you have already experienced it. For example, when you yawn, you may notice a kind of warmth or coolness flowing over your back to your head; sometimes you may get goose-pimples or tears in the eyes. A touch to the sole of the foot can have an effect on the whole body. When urinating, children often experience an involuntary shaking of the body. All of these are experiences of Qi.

If your body is shaken by icy coldness, that is a Qi movement. Also, the feeling that cold penetrates to the bones derives from movement of the Qi. It is well known that you get the common cold from exposure to cold temperatures. This can be explained by the movement of the Qi: the Qi retreats from the exposed parts of the body, and thus the immune system in those parts of the body, or the body as a whole, is weakened.

When you are excited, your heart pounds and you sweat. When you are embarrassed, you blush. When you have tender feelings, you get sexually excited. These are all caused by Qi-movement.

Acupuncture works by influencing the Qi at certain points on the body with a needle and subtle manual techniques. Other practices that have a perceptible effect on the flow and distribution of Qi include the use of herbs and other natural curative substances, Phytotherapy and *Tui Na-Anmo* curative massage, Acupressure, Moxibustion (treatments by means of burning Moxa-herb in direct proximity to acupuncture points), and Qigong exercises.

◆ What is Qigong?

"Gong" from the word "Qigong" has various meanings such as gain, achievement, performance, success, and efficacy. In combination with Qigong, it is an abbreviation for *Gongfu. Gongfu* means "time", "effort", "exertion", or "work." In an extended sense, it also means "ability" or "dexterity" acquired through time and effort. It designates abilities which are appropriated by bodily exercises, not only by intelligence and study. Many kinds of control of the body, such as dance and acrobatics, belong to *Gongfu,* including the skill of self-defense. Skills in the fighting arts are called *Wushu* in China.

Qigong thus means Gongfu of the Qi, or, the practice and study of influencing the Qi. It is also used to designate all of the exercises that are used to influence Qi. The word *Qigong* is as comprehensive as the word *music*. Because Qigong is the sum of an endless number of bodily experiences collected and developed over the ages, it embraces an incalculable number of individual exercises and curative methods, each of which bears its own name. Therefore, it is also spoken of as *Qigong Xue*, the science of Qigong.

Some Chinese dictionaries define Qigong as "breath exercise", but in Qigong, Qi is understood not only as breath, but in the same sense as in Chinese philosophy and medicine. Qi is the fundamental substance, or fundamental material, of the human body, of all living organisms, and of all life. In *Zhi Bei You*, one of the collections in *Zhuang Zi*, it is said: "Human life arises from the coming together of Qi; if it comes together there is life, and if it goes asunder, there is death." A proverb says: "Human beings live in the Qi as fish live in water. Qi is the root of human beings." (*Nan Jing*); "Human beings are in the Qi, Qi is in human beings." Humans are thus nothing other than "a part of the whole Qi in heaven and on earth" (*Bao Pu Zi* and *Tai Qing Tiao Qi Jing*).

In times past, the Chinese knew that the whole world arose from this Qi-Energy. Chinese philosophy and the Chinese view of the world are closely connected with this concept. Qi is, therefore, a frequently-used term, and expresses, besides its actual basic meaning, spiritual and moral strength. In other contexts it has additional meanings; for example: the Qi of the sky is the weather, the Qi of destiny is chance; to "stir up the Qi" means to be annoyed; the Qi of the public official is bureaucratic behavior.

♦ Properties of the Qi

Natural scientific research, for example in the realm of quantum physics, has shown that Qi, transmitted by various Qigong masters to other people, is a kind of electromagnetic wave with a very broad spectrum ranging from radio waves to micro-waves, infrared, visible light, ultra-violet, and radioactive waves. It can also possess the properties of infra-sound, or that of a magnetic field *(Qigong de Ke Xue Ji Chu)*.

The transmission of Qi to patients has already been achieved in China by Qigong masters (including Lin Hou Sheng, the Qigong master who also developed the 18 Figures in this book), who have successfully used it for anesthesia during thyroid operations.

◆ Where does Qi exist?

By means of Qigong exercises, practitioners located many Qi centers *(Dan Tian)* and Qi channels *(Mai)* in the human body. In addition there are many places, mostly on the Meridians, at which the Qi "enters or leaves" the body, and where the Qi allows itself to be influenced by internal and external forces. These places are designated in the West as acupuncture points—perhaps because acupuncture is best known in the West as Chinese therapy—although not all these points may be used in acupuncture.

Many of these points have an especially strong relationship with the external world. For this reason, they have names that refer to heavenly bodies such as "Sun and Moon" *(Ri-Yue)* or "Well of Heaven" *(Tian Jing)*, "Spring of Heaven" *(Tian-Quan)*, "Pond of Heaven" *(Tian-Chi)* or "Middle Pole" *(Zhong Ji)*. Many designations have connection with the weather: "Wind-Pond" *(Feng-Chi)*, "Wind-City" *(Feng-Shi)*, "Wind-Residence" *(Feng-Fu)*, "Cloud-Gate" *(Yun-Men)*, "Great-Thunder" *(Feng-Long)*, and "Crevice of Heaven" *(Lie-Que)*.

In addition, there are geographic designations such as "mountain", "valley", "hill"; designations for waters like "canal" or "river" *(Gou)*, "slough" *(Du)*, and "pond" *(Chi)*; and for dampness or a collection of water like "moor" or "swamp" *(Ze)*, "well" or "spring" *(Quan)*, and "sea" or "lake" *(Hai)*.

Many places owe their name to the function they exercise; for example, "palace" or "residence", "reservoir", "hall", "passage-way", "inner-court", "window", "gate", and "door."

Qi channels, (generally known as meridians) are systematically arranged to connect specific places of the body, and some of the meridians lead to internal organs. These latter meridians are often named after the respective organs, as in the liver-meridian, lung-meridian, heart-meridian, and so on. Other channels connect meridians with one another, and do not necessarily lead to organs. They have their own names, which are mostly given according to their function.

To put it another way, the Qi is distributed in our bodies, and enters and leaves through many places. The Qi permeates our bodies. Our bodies have contact with the environment and nature through the Qi. There is a continual exchange between our bodies (the microcosm), and nature (the macrocosm). Thus the Qi is in continuous movement in our bodies, both in the microcosm and the macrocosm.

◆ The Meridians (Jing Luo)

The Qi channels, or meridians, exist in the whole body, and form a network which links all the parts of the body together. This net is comparable to the streets of a city which intersect and connect different places (organs). The meridians are mostly arranged symmetrically in pairs of opposites.

Meridians and acupuncture points help to direct and to harmonize the Qi in your body, much as streets and connecting points in a city map help you to find your way. There are many theories about these Qi channels. It was first thought that the Qi channels corresponded with the nervous system because both systems have similar channels. But in time, it was discovered that the meridians have many routes where there are no corresponding nerve cords.

Moreover, the Qi does not flow like an electrical current. It flows more slowly, like the feeling that extends itself when you yawn or get goose-bumps.

In my opinion, the flow of the Qi has much to do with the body's musculature. I believe the Qi flows primarily in muscles, ligaments, tendons, and connective tissues. Many acupuncture and acupressure spots are found where the muscle fibers are most thickly bundled together, as well as at the beginning of muscles, ligaments, and tendons.

There is probably no specific anatomical structure that corresponds to the meridians. But this does not disprove the existence of meridians, because they are discerned by observation of the body. This is comparable to hearing a noise. You know that there are noises because you hear them. Even if you were not aware that noise is a movement of air and an oscillation of a specific frequency, you could not discover the nature of a noise. Similarly, for proof of the existence of meridians, no discovery of a specific anatomical structure is necessary.

Through thousands of years of research and experience, Qigong practitioners discovered the Qi centers, then individual meridians, and finally the entire meridian system.

By means of this knowledge of Qi centers and meridians, many methods of diagnosing and influencing the Qi have been developed. These methods include acupuncture and acupressure. Acupressure is known in Chinese as *Tui-Na, An-Mo,* and *Zhi-Zhen.* In Japanese, acupressure is called *Shiatsu. Shiatsu* and the various forms of acupressure use finger pressure for self-curative massage, and may also slap the body and rub the skin. There is also warming treatment (moxibustion) and traditional Chinese herbal and animal remedies. Finally, through the development of technology, some treatments use laser beams directed at acupuncture points.

For centuries Chinese Medicine has worked with success using both meridians and Qi. I think it would be a good idea if Western medicine were to examine the meridians scientifically. It would be a shame if the theory of meridians was rejected only because they have not yet been anatomically identified.

◆ Qi Centers (Dan Tian)

Dan means "medicine" in the form of pills. In conjunction with Qigong it has the meaning "pills of immortality," and takes its origin from Daoist Alchemy. *Tian* means "field" or "ground".

Dan Tian is the place where medicine for immortality grows. Thus, *Dan Tian* is a concept for many places where you concentrate when exercising, and where the Qi is collected. According to various dynasties, authors, and literary sources, there are hundreds of different expressions for the *Dan Tian*. There are, however, three primary locations: upper, middle, and lower *Dan Tian*.

In Qigong, if you speak of the *Dan Tian* without indicating its location, it is always the lower *Dan Tian*. There are different opinions about the exact location of the lower *Dan Tian:* from three centimeters below the navel to the genitals (thus perhaps the acupuncture points *Qi Hai, Guan Yuan* and *Shi Men*), or the acupuncture point *Hui Yin*, located between the external genitals and the anus.

The middle *Dan Tian* is usually recognized as the acupuncture point *Dan Zhong*, a spot on the breastbone near the nipples.

There are also differing opinions about the location of the upper Dan Tian. In the old days it was believed to be in the brain or the upper part of the head. Today it is generally assumed that the upper *Dan Tian* is an area inside the head between the eyebrows.

◆ Qi, Health, and Illness

You may have had the experience of feeling ill, yet the doctor was unable to make a diagnosis. The question is whether you were actually sick. If the answer was yes, why couldn't the doctor ascertain an illness? If no, why did you feel so weak and miserable? What does it mean if you feel pains and tensions which are considered harmless?

In order to understand what Qi has to do with health and sickness, and why Qigong is an effective therapeutic method, I will quote a statement from one of the oldest Chinese medical writings, *Huang Di Nei Jing:* "The wise heal that which is not yet sick."

"Not yet sick" means a Qi disturbance, a condition which could lead to an illness. In Chinese medicine, it is a matter of recognizing and removing the Qi disturbance as early as possible, before sickness can occur. For that purpose, you must concentrate more closely on Qi.

◆ The Two Primary Types of Qi

One can divide Qi into two primary types: the innate and the acquired.

Innate Qi is the Qi you have inherited from your parents. Traditionally it is designated as the Qi from heaven and earth. It is your original Qi (*Yuan Qi*, 元氣 or *Qi* 炁), your basic life-energy.

The Japanese, who early in their history used Chinese ideograms almost exclusively, used the word "original Qi" or *Yuan Qi* to mean "health." Instead of asking "How are you?" a Japanese person would ask, "How is your Yuan Qi?" As you can see from this example, the value of the innate Qi is of fundamental importance to the ancient Chinese and Japanese people.

Acquired Qi is the Qi you take in from birth onward through eating, drinking, and breathing. It is the energy that comes from outside your body, from Heaven (air) and Earth (food). The acquired Qi gives you the energy necessary to maintain your general life functions. The quality of your food and air, the kind and manner of breathing, and your lifestyle plays an important role in determining the quality of this Qi condition. Finally, the acquired Qi also influences the innate Qi in mental and physical ways.

The innate Qi has its place in a system designated as the "kidneys." This system embraces not only the named organ in the anatomical sense, but also the pertinent meridian with its corresponding anatomical structures and a large functional area which makes itself felt in physical as well as in mental ways.

According to Chinese medicine, the innate Qi is guided through the kidneys up to the stomach-spleen system. There it binds itself with the Qi acquired through nourishment. It rises to the lung system, and encounters the clear Qi which is breathed in by the lungs. Our actual Qi is the sum of these three. The innate Qi determines the original duration of your life and your original state of health. The acquired Qi works with the innate Qi so that the two kinds together determine both the actual state of your health and the actual duration of your life. If the Qi is harmonious, you are healthy; if it is in disharmony, you are ill. If an aggravated disharmony becomes chronic, the innate Qi can be so quickly consumed that life ends prematurely.

◆ The Five Physiological Functions of Qi

Qi has essentially five physiological functions:

1. *Driving force*

Qi is a very active, fine substance which affects the growth and development of the body, and the physiological activities of all its organs, and allows blood and other bodily fluids to generate, be correctly distributed, excrete, and flow. If the Qi is too weak, it is called *Xu* which means "inadequate", "exhausted", or "empty". It means the blood and other bodily fluids are no longer produced in sufficient quantities. They circulate more slowly, or remain immobile, and corresponding illnesses develop.

2. *Source of Warmth*

Qi provides the human body with constant warmth. In this way, it maintains the condition of the blood and other bodily fluids and enables all the organs to function properly. When the Qi is not able to fulfill this task adequately, the body temperature sinks. Some parts of the body (such as the hands and feet) become colder. Bodily fluids flow more slowly, which is known as *Han Zheng* (symptoms of illness caused by cold).

3. *Resistance/Prevention*

The Qi protects the body against negative external influences, such as extreme heat and cold. It also combats illnesses which have already attacked the body. When the Qi is weakened, the power of resistance is insufficient. You become more susceptible to illness, and require a longer period to regain your health.

4. *Stabilization and Care* (Gu *and* Sche)

Gu means "to stabilize" and "to strengthen." *Sche* has the meaning "to absorb" or "to care for." Qi maintains, for example, the good condition of the blood and other bodily fluids, and prevents their loss. It sees that the blood does not leave its vessels. Qi is responsible for the discharge of, among others, sweat, urine, saliva, digestive juice, and semen. If something is wrong with the Qi, it can cause inexplicable sweating, premature ejaculation, wet dreams, constant loss of saliva, or incontinence. Together with the driving force (the first function), *Gu* and *Sche* direct the origin of the bodily fluids, their movement, distribution, their preservation, and their secretion.

5. *Transformation* (Qi Hua)

Qi Hua is a concept from Traditional Chinese Medicine, and means "change" and "transformation" by means of Qi. Concretely, it means all metabolic occurrences by which the fine substances ingested at feeding are transformed into blood and other bodily fluids, and by which acquired Qi arises. It accepts the useful substances, and excretes the rest. If it does not function properly, the taking in of nourishment, metabolism, digestion, and secretion are impaired, and corresponding illnesses arise.

In all five functions, Qi is necessary for life, and its absence causes illnesses.

◆ Qi, Body, and Mind

For various reasons, the Qi can fall into disorder. Thus in *Huang Di Nei Jing* it reads: "Hundreds (all) of illnesses arise through Qi disharmony. When one is angry, the Qi rises through the body; with joy it flows easily; with sadness the Qi is despondent; with anxiety the Qi falls or is weakened; in coldness it draws back, and in heat it escapes; with fright the Qi falls into confusion; with bodily overwork, it is used up; with too much reflection and musing, it is blocked up. These are several reasons for the confusion of Qi."

According to the theory of Traditional Chinese Medicine, anger damages the liver, too much joy and laughter damage the heart, too much thinking and reflection affect the spleen and stomach, too much sadness and weeping affect the lungs, and anxiety damages the kidneys. This theory corresponds to a psychosomatic explanation of the change in organs, and the origin of disease.

When the Qi is in harmony it is designated as *Qi He*. When the Qi is in disorder, you may be said to be suffering from negative influences, or a bad Qi condition. In earlier times it was called "demonic influences" or "evil Qi" (*Xie Qi*). A bad Qi condition leads first to feelings of discomfort, then to pain, and in further development, to functional disturbances or organic changes. This is how illnesses arise. Thus the advice: in order to heal the preliminary stage of an illness, you must learn the Qi and its nature, and bring a disturbed Qi condition back into harmony.

Chinese medicine does not purposely speak of the psychosomatic. Chinese medicine, which embraces the unity of body and psyche, is in itself already psycho-somatic medicine. Qi influences the body and mind, and in turn is influenced by them. This can be illustrated as Body↔Qi↔Mind/Psyche.

In order to make this point clear, compare your body to a radio. The radio produces a sound which you can hear reasonably well. This corresponds to your mind, or psyche. If the radio is functioning properly, then the sound is good.

Of course the radio needs energy, such as batteries, to make it work. This is comparable to Qi. When the radio is working correctly, it uses little energy, and yet produces a good sound. That corresponds to a properly-functioning body with a well-balanced psyche.

When mental or emotional burdens such as sadness, annoyance, stress, or anxiety appear, the Qi harmony is disturbed. This corresponds to a radio that is constantly too loud. Not only does it use more energy so that the batteries are prematurely depleted, but the sound also becomes poorer, and finally the radio stops functioning. In the human body, the Qi is disturbed by different mental burdens, and its flow is hindered. As a result, psychosomatic symptoms such as pain, tension, or ulcers appear in the body.

If your body is burdened by physical overwork, excessive sexual activity, poor nutrition and posture, or even injuries, the Qi is also harmed. Not only do tiredness and physical complaints come to the fore, but so do mental and spiritual impairments such as nervousness, feverish activity, irritability, and other psychic manifestations of illness.

Qi is like water in a basin. If the basin is full, you are healthy. The consumption of energy through physical and mental burdens is like water flowing out of the basin. When the Qi is no longer sufficiently present, health deteriorates, and you become susceptible to illness. In order to remain well, as much water must flow in as flows out. A balanced proportion must always remain. You can replenish the Qi with a healthy diet, physical activities, and Qigong exercises. But you can also lessen the demand on the Qi by keeping physical and mental demands to a minimum.

In my opinion, most chronic illnesses are of a psychosomatic Qigong nature, and can be cured by restoration of the Qi harmony. That is what both Traditional Chinese Medicine and Qigong do. Even very advanced cancer illnesses have been cured by Qigong therapy. No "miracle" needs occur in order to heal such illnesses because the illnesses did not occur by a "miracle."

You need to care for your own health. You cannot burden your body and mind at will in order to "enjoy" life. It is also not the fault of the doctors when a very advanced illness can no longer be cured. You are responsible for your own health. It is not the task of the doctor to say: "Live it up and don't be concerned about your health. If you get sick we'll be there." You do not get ill (in the passive sense)—you create the conditions that allow illness to arise.

◆ The History and Schools of Qigong

Qigong exercises existed before the word Qigong, and it is difficult to say how old Qigong really is. Perhaps it is as old as the human race, because it was not "invented" at a specific time, but gradually developed by observation of the body and its reactions. As a more or less systematic exercise and healing method , Qigong is probably 4000 years old, and possibly even 7000 years old.

The bodily experiences that gave rise to Qigong still exist today. If you are tired, for example, you yawn, stretch your arms, and expand or turn your body. Thereafter you feel relaxed and refreshed. Or you may sit down, close your eyes, and breathe more quietly in order to reinvigorate yourself. This is the origin of stretching and expansion exercises, and concentration exercises without bodily movements (*Jing Gong* or static exercises).

If you feel a tension or a heavy pain in some part of your body, you might pat the area gently with the palm, or rub or press it with a finger so that the unpleasant feeling subsides. This is the origin of self-healing massage.

If you are depressed or sad, sometimes you sigh deeply. That is the natural starting point for exercises that developed later—for example, the healing sounds which are used for the treatment of many illnesses of the internal organs.

In *Huang Di Nei Jing*, it is mentioned that in the middle region of China where it is naturally damp and the soil is thus productive, the population had access to an abundance of different foods without much work. Thus they suffered from many health problems resulting from lack of movement after luxurious dining. To counter these health problems, sequences of exercises were developed such as *Dao-Yin* ("lead" and "direct") and *An-Qiao* ("press the palm" and "flex the foot"). These are techniques to activate and direct the Qi in the body, and to harmonize the Qi through self-healing massage. These are the original forms of Qigong exercises, which later were developed into definite patterns of movements.

In many other classical works, it is stated that some 4,000 years ago, in the Tang-Yao-period in the central regions of China (around the middle and lower courses of the Yellow River) the population was plagued by numerous illnesses of the skin, muscles, and joints. They developed *Wu* (dance, jumping, and hopping). This was a set of complete exercises, with the help of which they trained the whole mechanism of movement, and increased the blood supply.

From a painted bowl approximately 5,000 years old, excavated in the province of Qinghai, it was discovered that people at that time already exercised Qigong together in a kind of dance. Another form of bodily movement developed from the imitation of animal movements. All these were original forms of Qigong exercises utilizing bodily movements (*Dong Gong* or exercises with body movements).

Qigong embraces many schools, but at least five main trends have been identified:

1. The Daoist School.

2. The Buddhist School, whose exercises were brought, in part, with Buddhism from India to China, and carried over to Japan. In this way, many Yoga exercises have come to China, and were integrated there in a school which shows some similarities to Yoga. Chinese Buddhists also independently developed some Qigong exercises.

3. The Confucian School.

4. The medical school, which created a multiplicity of therapeutic exercises that are still being developed today, and are used in hospital treatments.

5. The *Wushu (Gongfu* or *Kung Fu)* School, whose exercises were developed by martial artists in order to strengthen the body and promote the harmony of body and spirit.

Qigong exercises can also be divided into "soft" and "hard." Hard Qigong was developed mainly by martial artists to make the body invulnerable to blows and strikes. Practitioners of hard Qigong are able to bore through a brick with a finger, or break a grave-stone with a head thrust without getting hurt. There are many other examples, and although hard Qigong contributes to the stabilization of spirit and body, this book focuses essentially on soft Qigong. In spite of these divisions, everything is included under the concept of Qigong.

Taijiquan (old transcription: *T'ai Chi Ch'uan)* is, briefly, an exercise derived from Qigong. Qigong is the collective concept for all forms of exercise directed by the principle of body, breath, and spirit. If we compare the concept of Qigong with music, *Taijiquan* corresponds to a symphony. *Taijiquan* belongs to the Qigong School of *Wushu (Gongfu).* According to its name, it also belongs to the Daoist school, because *Taiji* is a concept derived from Chinese philosophy. It has a meaning of *Yi:* the origin of everything, the world-beginning balance of *Yin* and *Yang* (harmony). *Taiji* is also interpreted as the truth of all things between heaven and earth, or as Qi that existed before the separation of heaven and earth when the world arose out of chaos, still clear, empty, and void (Chinese: *Hun-Dun, Qing Xu*). *Quan* means "fist." *Taijiquan* is thus the art of self-defense by means of bare hands according to the *Yin-Yang* harmony of *Taiji*.

CHAPTER 2

Qigong
The Foundations

◆ The Qigong Principle

There are three essential elements in Qigong exercises:

1. The body *(Shen)*, meaning body posture and body movement for achieving relaxation and leading the Qi.

2. The breath *(Xi)*, meaning breathing techniques.

3. The heart *(Xin)*, meaning concentration and visualization. The Chinese character for the heart means not only the physical organ, but the reflective level of the mind.

The Body (Shen)

Qigong can be practiced standing, sitting, or lying down. It can be performed statically *(Jing-Gong)* or dynamically *(Dong-Gong)*, or, of course, both statically and dynamically. The correct body stance and posture is a precondition for the right proportion of tension and relaxation, and for activating and leading the Qi.

The Breath (Xi)

There are many techniques for breathing, which have been developed from bodily experiences. For example, there is chest breathing, abdominal breathing, and mixed breathing (chest and abdomen). Several techniques exist for abdominal breathing: for example, natural and "reverse" abdominal breathing. In natural abdominal breathing, the lower abdomen expands when inhaling. In "reverse" abdominal breathing the lower abdomen is drawn in by inhalation, and expanded by exhalation. Another technique is known as skin-breathing or embryo breathing, which is also designated by some as "no-breathing" *(Wu-Xi),* because the process of breathing is no longer perceptible: even down-feathers can no longer be moved by such breathing. In this technique the skin probably takes over the main work of breathing. Moreover, metabolism is slowed down so much that very little oxygen is needed. Breathing techniques for hard Qigong are not presented here; they can be found in the appropriate instruction manuals.

The Heart (Xin)

Xin refers to concentration on the body, its movements, and breathing. It is, more-over, a kind of observation of the Qi, its movements and surroundings. During Qigong exercise you should be aware of what occurs in the body and what sensations may develop; for example, a feeling of cold or warmth.

Visualization can be a support when exercising. You can imagine that you are in a lovely natural environment, breathing fresh air, and have no cares. It is a matter of intu-itive, positive attitudes toward exercise. If you have ailments or are sick, you can imag-ine that by exercise the ailments will be relieved or the sickness cured. Also, in the meridian system, visualization serves to set the Qi in motion through corresponding thoughts or motions through channels in the body.

These three elements of Qigong are in constant, reciprocal action. Without the cor-rect body posture, you cannot breathe properly because movements of the body, such as expanding the chest cavity, and movement of the diaphragm, makes breathing possi-ble. By means of the right breathing technique, you can relax the body and so guide the Qi easily through the body. But in order to find the correct positions and movements of the body, as well as appropriate breathing techniques, you need concentration. You must exercise, at the same time, on the mental and physical levels.

The correct breathing technique also influences your concentration and imagina-tion. If, for example, your breathing is hectic, strenuous, and irregular, your heart begins to work more quickly. You will become excited, nervous, and hence, distracted.

These three elements are equally important, and not one should be neglected.

What is the Difference Between Qigong, Gymnastics, and Sport?

On the basis of the three elements of the body, the breath, and the heart (mind), you can see the difference between Qigong and other forms of sport such as dance or gym-nastics. To be sure, Qigong sometimes involves bodily movements, and appears at times as a gentle dance. Yet in dancing the body moves to express something. The purpose of gymnastics is to relax parts of the body and to train the muscles. With Qigong, the pur-pose of movement is to enable the Qi to flow through the body. Focus is directed not only on the physical movements, but still more on the Qi actually flowing through the body. Qigong is not merely the imitation of movements without knowledge of their significance. Hence, you should always know what purpose the movement has, and what visualization it is connected with. Only when the exercises are performed in accordance with these essentials are they Qigong exercises. Without the body, breath, and heart (mind), the effects cannot properly be manifested, even though the movements appear to be correct and there are some pleasant and refreshing effects.

What Is the Difference Between Qigong and Autogenous Training?

The goal of autogenous training is to soothe and to relax the body through concentration. A practitioner attempts to regulate the breathing, slow the heart beat, and warm the hands, feet, and other parts of the body. The goal of Qigong is to guide the Qi consciously through the body. Where autogenous training stops, Qigong rightly begins.

◆ Further Basic Parts of Qigong

Qigong practice includes preparatory, main, and concluding exercises, self-curative massage, knowledge of correct Qigong practice, and a healthy life-style.

Preparatory Exercises

Preparatory exercises such as warming up and stretching are a part of Qigong practice. By means of Qigong, the Qi should flow through the body. Warm-up exercises help to set the Qi in motion. An example is tapping, in which you tap specific body parts either with hands or with an object, to stimulate the circulation of the blood. Furthermore, there are stretching exercises which activate the joints and the stimulate the meridians. If the joints are warm and loose, and the meridians stimulated, the Qi can flow better in these places. Some kinds of preparatory exercises also help you concentrate and relax. Stretching is recommended for all Qigong exercises.

Concluding Exercises

Concluding exercises are of great importance for Qigong in order to bring the activation of the Qi to a gentle close. Because the Qi is guided and collected in the body by means of external and internal movements, as well as by various kinds of concentration, it is beneficial to bring the Qi, and thus the body, back to its normal condition. The Qi should be correctly distributed in the body. The sudden ending of an exercise can result in discomfort and have other serious consequences because the Qi is suddenly stopped or blocked. It is similar to feeling unwell or unbalanced when suddenly torn from a deep sleep, but it can be even more unpleasant if you stop a serious Qigong routine without a concluding exercise. Therefore, it is said by experts: "Even if the sky caves in, there must be a final exercise."

If for any reason you are unable to make a concluding exercise during your practice, you should return to a Qigong condition as soon as you can. Then, exercise as deeply as possible, and then slowly and as intensely as possible, make a final exercise until you sense a feeling of harmony. You may need several repetitions of the whole procedure to achieve that feeling.

Self-Healing Massage

Qigong exercises include self-curative massage and acupressure, because they are also methods of activating the Qi in the body.

Self-curative massage involves tapping and rubbing the body's surface. Circulation is thus improved, and the Qi activated. With specific methods the Qi is also guided through the body in correspondence to the meridian system. Self-curative massage can be a very useful accompaniment to other Qigong exercises, but also can be used independently.

Acupressure denotes a series of special techniques from China by which pressure is applied with the hand, mainly with the tips of the thumbs, to stimulate specific areas of the body, especially "acupuncture points." By this means, the Qi is also influenced and guided.

Necessary Knowledge for the Practice of Qigong

Since Qigong is quite different from other kinds of exercise, it is not sufficient only to know how to do the movements. You must also know the right time to exercise, the duration of the exercise, and possible sources of error.

Healthy Life Style

Qigong begins with a healthy life style. It is not just practical daily exercise, but a conscious, healthy style of living. The main goal of Qigong is to produce a state of Qi harmony and a stability that embraces spirit and body. You should live consciously and continuously according to Qi principles. In everything you do—reading, walking, eating, speaking, working, etc.—you should pay attention to your body, attempt to improve your posture, and to move and breathe harmoniously. This alone can bring positive results because the Qi is activated and harmonized.

CHAPTER 3

Qigong
Practice

A) DO's AND DON'Ts

◆ When To Practice

Generally, you can practice Qigong at any time of the day. But because the Qi in the macrocosm influences your microcosm, there are times of the day that are especially suitable for certain exercise. There are four time periods especially important for the course of the Qi: noon, midnight, morning, and evening. Morning means the hours between 5 and 7 A.M. and evening means between 5 and 7 P.M. These times correspond to sunrise and sunset in China. Noon and midnight are the times between 11–1 P.M. and 11–1 A.M. respectively, and are the times in which Yin and Yang reach their high points and begin to transform themselves into their opposites. If you have a routine job, practice is recommended in the morning, at night before going to sleep, and sometime during the day.

You should not exercise on either an empty stomach or after a full meal. In Qigong exercise, stomach juices increase, hormones become depleted, different parts of the body have increased blood supply according to flow of the Qi, and stomach-intestinal movements occur. If you regularly practice when hungry, stomach trouble is possible.

Qi is the "ruler of the blood," and where Qi flows, the blood is also directed. After eating, the digestive system uses considerable blood. Therefore, you should not, with Qigong exercises, lead the Qi (and hence the blood) to the body's extremities, because this will disrupt the digestive process.

As a rule, you should not exercise an hour before or after eating. Through experience you will discover for yourself how full your stomach can be in order to exercise comfortably.

If you exercise in the morning after waking up, do not have a full breakfast or drink strong coffee or alcohol. You can, however, have liquids because liquids stimulate stomach-intestine movement, and serve as an "internal massage." This massage supports Qigong exercises. In China, it is common to eat a little rice broth or noodle soup, or drink lukewarm water with dissolved honey before morning practice. Honey stills the hunger and provides for sufficient blood sugar, which prevents dizziness. A clear head is very important during Qigong for mental concentration and the auto-suggestive power of imagination and visualization.

It is very beneficial to exercise in the morning between 5 and 7 (later in winter, earlier in summer). With the rising sun, nature awakens and you can take up its positive influences. Morning is a very effective time for Qigong exercise.

Practice around mid-day is controversial among Qigong experts in China. There are definite exercises designed specifically for mid-day. Unless an exercise is clearly stated as being for mid-day, you should avoid Qigong practice between 11 A.M. and 1 P.M.

The setting of the sun is also a time when nature has great influence on your body. In the countryside you can easily see that the birds are very active at this time, as they are in the morning. In the city there is traffic at this time, the air is polluted, and it is noisy, which makes the early evening less suitable for exercise. You should do your best to avoid areas congested with air and noise pollution during evening practice. In the country however, in the nature and good air, you can exercise wonderfully at this time. Of course, take care not to have an empty or a full stomach.

Midnight is a special time for Qigong exercise, especially Still Qigong *(Jing Gong)*. It is a transition to the new day. This is a time when everything is quietest, and in great harmony. Thereafter, nature arises again, as well as the Qi. Thus, you can concentrate clearly and relax at this time. Some people also work best, and with mental concentration, at night. But for those with day jobs, this time is, of course, unsatisfactory. You should not force yourself to stay awake or get up from sleep for midnight practice. Instead, exercise in the evening before going to bed.

Qigong exercise before sleep is especially important because you have burdened your spirit and body throughout the day with work. Before going to bed, where you will remain for hours in the same condition, you should relax your body and spirit. Then you can sleep more quietly, and recover better. Some people believe that because they have so little time for sleep, they would rather go right to bed. It is better, however, to use half an hour before sleeping for Qigong rather than to prolong a restless sleep, because the body's recovery begins when exercising with Qigong.

At certain times of the day the macrocosm especially influences specific organs in your body, the microcosm. Therefore, appropriate exercises have been developed for specific organ systems at specific times of the day.

◆ When not to Exercise

You should not exercise during bad weather, heavy fog, storm or hail, solar and lunar eclipses, great heat, thunderstorms, or when a thunderstorm approaches. Exercise is a process by which good influences from the macrocosm are assimilated. In the above-mentioned weather conditions, nature itself is not balanced. If the storm is past, the air fresh, and nature balanced, you can then exercise again.

Women who are menstruating should only practice Qigong exercises specifically designed for the menstruation cycle. They should, however, pay attention to whether the exercise has a negative effect, and if so, stop immediately. If they feel well, they can continue to exercise.

Special care is required with Qigong during pregnancy. Like menstruation, only specific exercises should be performed.

◆ Where to Practice

You should be undisturbed during Qigong practice to help maintain a concentrated mind. Find a place where you will not be disturbed by telephone calls, passers-by, or other distractions. Surroundings are also important. The best place is a quiet spot in the open air surrounded by suitable plants or trees. Practicing indoors is also acceptable.

Many plants have a good influence on the body, especially conifers *(Song Shu)*. *Song* denotes a species of conifer, and also means in contemporary Chinese, "loose, relaxed". The Qi from this kind of tree has an especially relaxing and quieting effect. When walking in a coniferous forest you may experience easy breathing and very refreshing air. From their needles you can perceive very positive Qi and incorporate it. Trees with leaves, such as maples and weeping willows, are also very helpful.

The proximity of some plants, for example, Oleander, should be avoided when exercising. Oleander is known to be poisonous, and has a very tense Qi, which can only have negative influences. But not all poisonous plants have bad Qi. You must discover from your own experience which plants feel relaxing and harmonious. Sensitivity to the Qi of plants varies according to the person. Oleander is not only poisonous and contains bad Qi, but can even cause pain.

I started to practice Qigong as a child. My master always said that I should seek proximity of lovely flowers and large old trees, so I exercised one summer evening before a splendid oleander. When I noticed pains in my lower arms, I made a concluding exercise. Because the pains continued, I asked my master to explain their cause. He asked me what kind of plants I had exercised near. When I replied, "near an oleander" the matter was clear to him. Oleander is not suitable for Qigong exercise and the pains resulted from this. The pain in the lower arms, wrists, and finger continued for a week. The pain sat deeply in my bones and to drain it off I had to exercise for a few days.

Good surroundings are mountains, oceans, rivers, and generally all bodies of water, and where the air is clear and moist. A newly mown meadow is especially recommended because the Qi is still very strong.

During exercise in fresh air, your warmed up body should not cool off. You can exercise outdoors in the winter if you keep your body warm with appropriate clothing. Whenever exercising in the open, be sure not to be exposed too much to the wind, especially from behind.

◆ **What to Wear**

In general, there are no rules regarding clothing. But since relaxation has fundamental importance for Qigong, it is best to wear comfortable and loose-fitting clothes. Clothing made from natural materials such as cotton or silk is best. Sneakers or athletic shoes are recommended, but shoes with flat heels are also suitable.

Do not wear jewelry and watches when exercising. They can disturb the effectiveness of the exercise. If you wear these accessories regularly, you are no longer conscious of their influence. After you have exercised a long time without jewelry or a watch, you can ascertain if they impair your Qigong practice, and accordingly wear or remove them.

If you wear uncomfortable clothing constantly, you may no longer notice that they can produce nervousness and tension. If you cannot wear comfortable clothing, for example, at work, and you want to practice Qigong, loosen your collar and tie, your belt and/or waistband, and remove high-heeled shoes.

Whatever clothing you choose to exercise in, it should not to be tight around the waist, because the Qi needs to flow easily to make the exercise most effective.

◆ **Eating and Drinking**

Before exercising, you should ingest little which has an influence on consciousness—for example, alcohol, coffee, or tea—even if you are accustomed to the effects of the beverage. For Qigong exercise you need a clear head. If your consciousness and thoughts are affected by alcohol, or even by strong coffee or tea, concentration suffers. If you are not calm or relaxed, the exercise is impaired. This is also true for the after-effects of an evening with a lot of alcohol.

Effects of strong drinks vary from person to person. Thus, there are those who can enjoy much within limits and practice Qigong, if they have the feeling that both can be enjoyed. If you cannot enjoy both, you must decide whether to drink alcohol or strong coffee, or to practice Qigong seriously. If you have gained body sensitivity by means of Qigong exercises, you will sense how important concentration is, and how easily it can be disturbed by delightful poisons.

◆ Duration of Qigong Exercises

There are Qigong exercises of fixed duration, and exercises whose duration is up to you. The standing exercise in this book can take hours, or only fifteen minutes. On the whole, no fixed duration is recommended, but beginners should do the exercises until they experience effects. Beginners generally need more time to relax and regulate the body and mind and feel the Qi, and exercises that are too brief will not provide sufficient time for this. Only when you have regulated the body's bearing and carriage according to the Qigong principle can Qi flow easily through the body, and the benefits of Qigong practice be realized.

In the beginning you should practice daily, at least long enough to reach a deep meditative state and remain in this Qigong condition for a time that is comfortable. For beginners, an exercise period of 15 to 30 minutes is recommended in order to learn to relax the body and regulate its bearing and carriage.

◆ How Long Does the Effect of a Qigong Exercise Last?

The effect of a Qigong exercise cannot, of course, be compared with that of a medication which has a specific time of effectiveness. With medications the results depend on their dispersal in the body, the biochemical processes of exhaustion or elimination, and body weight.

Qigong works because the Qi is brought into order, and body and spirit are in a condition of harmony. In this condition the body cannot become ill or, if it is already ill because of disturbed Qi, it can become healthy again through restoration of harmony.

This harmony can be disturbed if you behave in an unhealthy way; for example, if immediately after the completion of the final exercise you argue, get exited or annoyed, or engage in strenuous physical activity.

Immediately after Qigong exercise, you should not go to the toilet because urination and defecation bring the Qi into definite motion. By means of the exercise you have just attained a higher level of Qi harmony, which should not be disturbed unnecessarily. Do not restrain yourself from going to the bathroom during or after Qigong practice because this tension is inconducive to Qigong exercise. However, it is best to use the toilet beforehand.

The Qi must be cared for after the concluding exercise, and harmony be maintained as long as possible. So long as the Qi harmony is maintained, the exercise has continuing effect. However, you should not over-exercise. The exercises have no effects if you are exhausted and cannot concentrate.

Qigong is not a miraculous medicine that you take in order to avoid paying attention to your health. Qigong is thus not an exercise with an effect over a specific period of time, but a way of living which should be cultivated 24 hours a day.

When an exercise is to be done twice a day, it is correspondingly less effective if you can do it only once. If you practice more often than prescribed, no "overdose" results. On the contrary, the exercises have a more intense effect.

However, you should not force yourself to exercise, but only exercise if in the proper mood, because otherwise the necessary concentration may be lacking.

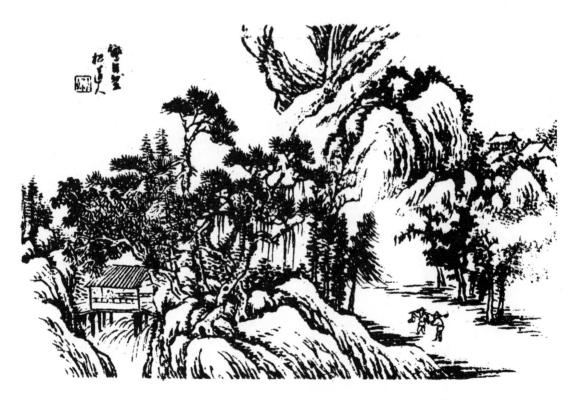

Reproduction of a drawing from the Qing dynasty, circa 1670 A.D.

B) QIGONG

♦ Standing Exercise

With this exercise you will learn the basic posture for almost all Qigong exercises.

Your feet should be parallel and approximately shoulder-width apart. Distribute your weight evenly on the soles of your feet so that there is a very firm and deep connection with the ground, as if your feet were rooted. Let your feet become heavy and warm, and feel your connection to the ground pass up through the soles to the legs and throughout your entire body.

Maintain this feeling and then turn your attention to your body, the highest point of which is called *Bai Hui,* located at the top of the head (Please see pg. 119 for the location of the *Bai Hui,* which is marked with a 'Δ'). Your head should rest easily on the spinal cord. Tuck in your chin somewhat. Look straight ahead. Beginners are advised to close their eyes gently, in order not to be distracted. Your head should now form a straight line with the spine. Imagine that each cervical vertebra is placed one on another in the air.

Your face should be relaxed as well as your shoulders. To help relax the shoulders, you can consciously raise and stretch them when inhaling, and drop them when exhaling. Repeat this process several times. Be sure that your shoulders drop in a relaxed way, and do not "force" them downward.

The chest should not be forced outward, but also not pulled in. The idea of "chest out, stomach in" does not apply here.

Turn your mind to your arm pits, and create a space there while allowing the shoulder blades to part without exertion. Imagine that an opening appears between the shoulder blades. At the same time, rotate the upper arms slightly inward so that the bending sides face your body. Your hands are loose beside the body, hanging from the upper arms, and your palms face your body.

Next, raise your pelvis slightly by pushing the lower part a bit forward and retracting the upper part. At the same time, loosen your stomach muscles. The area between the hips and pelvis should not be tense. By means of raising the pelvis you compensate for curvature of the lumbar spinal column, and open up the lower back area (about to the height of the kidneys). Tensions and weakness often predominate in this area, and cause pains, which can eventually lead to damage of the spinal disks and vertebrae. Chinese medicine, therefore, considers this area very important, and calls a point in that area the "gate of life" *(Mingmen)* or "the most important flash" *(Yao).*

The hips and posterior muscles should be relaxed. Next, bend the knees gently and assume a position as if you are sitting in a saddle. This strains the upper thigh a bit. The tension should not, however be too strong, especially for beginners. The knees should stay over the feet, and not extend beyond the toes. Imagine that the legs form an arch, and you assume the position of a rider. Draw the knees a bit apart, so that the lower legs, as seen from the front, stand vertically. Take care that your body weight is distributed evenly on the soles of the feet, and that the weight is not displaced on the outer edges. For that purpose a certain tension in the ankle joint is sometimes necessary, in order to guarantee a stable position. Even weight distribution on the soles of the feet can be maintained if you periodically check and correct the position of all parts of the body. To test if the balls of the feet or the heels are carrying more weight, rock back and forth in the ankle joints. If the weight feels uneven, find a neutral point between balls and heels for uniform distribution. To take a rest, consciously placing more weight on the balls or the heels of your feet is allowed.

In this posture you learn to employ as little force as possible to remain standing, and to feel no great effort. Direct your concentration on maintaining correct posture, and at the same time breathe naturally and without effort and excitement, and relax the entire body as much as possible. Your relaxed face should smile easily. If it is difficult, you are not yet physically or psychologically relaxed. Unnecessary tension consumes energy, and causes nervousness and cramps which negatively influence relaxation. That is true for almost all Qigong exercises. Thus, you must always be able to smile without strain. Also, a concluding exercise is necessary for ending the standing exercise.

Smiling does not mean tensing the mimetic muscular system, such as drawing the corners of the mouth upwards. Smiling comes from within. Anyone who is sad, looks sad; anyone who is happy can smile easily; and anyone whose body is tense cannot appear happy. Thus, you can read from a smile whether the body is relaxed.

If you do not succeed in relaxing the face, it is an indication that the body is cramped. Then you should try once more, step by step, to relax completely. When the body is relaxed, smiling occurs because the face shows the condition of the whole body.

If you are happy and laugh, your whole body laughs, even the inner organs. In German one says, "my heart is laughing." Internal organs are always affected by psychological burdens. The face is only a visible part of the unity of your body and spirit, and can show moods more clearly than other parts of the body.

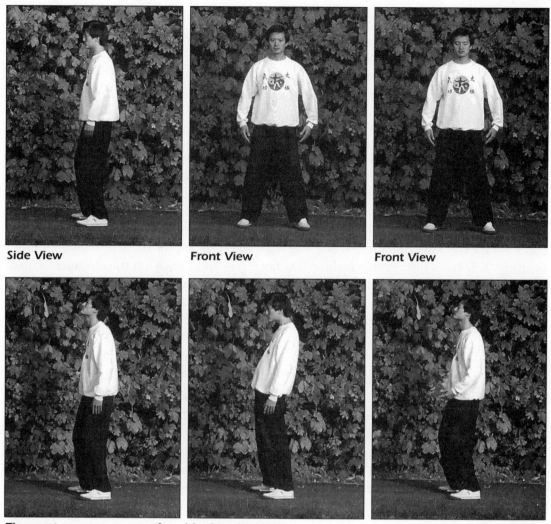

Side View   Front View   Front View

The most common errors of positioning the body

◆ CONCLUDING EXERCISES

These concluding exercises are to be done at the end of meditation and the 18 Figures. They are demonstrated before the 18 Figures because they are essential to your Qigong practice and should not be left out. Become familiar with these movements and always remember to perform a concluding exercise after your Qigong practice.

Concluding Exercise 1:

Stand in the basic position described above. The body should again be awakened. Lift your hands and slowly stretch the arms in order to embrace the cosmos, the positive Qi, to take up good influences from the macrocosm, and to guide them into the *Dan Tian,* about two inches below your navel. Draw your hands slowly together, one over the other, and place them on your stomach beneath the navel. Men should place the left hand flat on the lower abdomen, and the right hand on top of the left; women should position their hands in reverse fashion. Do not press too tightly on the stomach. Those who are trained, do it in such a way that the hands barely touch one another and the stomach. After a few breaths, move your hands slowly out to the sides of the body, without moving Qi from the body. Repeat this procedure three or more times. Movements do not have to be synchronized with breathing; that is, a single movement can quietly last for several breaths. But it is better if you start to raise your hands when inhaling, and after several breaths, direct your hands to the *Dan Tian* (lower abdomen) when exhaling.

During the entire procedure, imagine that you have called all positive Qi from outside and from within, and are bringing it to the center in the lower abdomen. After you have collected the Qi at least three times, open your eyes and make relaxed fists (with the palms facing the body) and let them hang at your sides. Remain standing quietly for a few minutes, become alert, and direct your consciousness to its normal condition. Finally, draw your left foot back and close your legs.

After the conclusion of a Qigong exercise, you should not immediately engage in activity, or burden the body excessively, but remain quiet for a time, perhaps for 30 minutes, so that the body can actually take up the collected Qi and preserve its harmony. This is similar to the need for a time of digestion after eating.

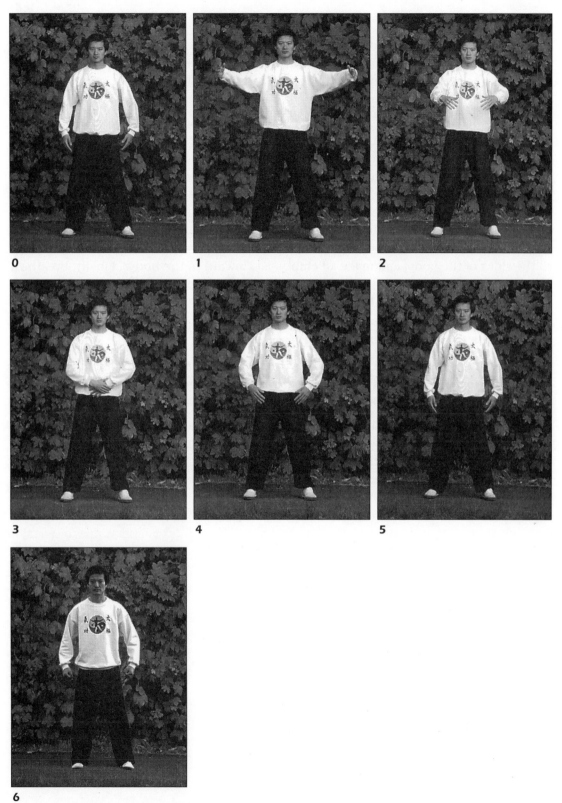

0

1

2

3

4

5

6

Concluding Exercise 2:

The exercise represents a more comprehensive version of Concluding Exercise 1. After the first two embraces in Example 1, you can also make an embrace from behind. For that purpose, again allow the hands to drop slowly to the side after placing them together on the pelvis for the second time.

When inhaling, you now draw your hands behind your back. The palms are first drawn behind and gradually towards the body, as if you were holding a pillow in front of the kidney area. Imagine that the palms are "suns" which radiate warmth. The body is calm and relaxed. Breathe naturally and guide the positive Qi through the kidneys and lumbar muscles to the body. Then move your palms to the front of your body along the belt line, place them on top of each other and then on the lower abdomen below the navel *(Dan Tian)*. Imagine that the entire belt-line is relaxed and warm. Remain with these thoughts for a few breaths—perhaps a minute—then let the hands carefully drop to the sides of the body, and make an empty fist (inward to the body). Finally, breathe a few times naturally and deeply, open your eyes, and remain standing for a while. Then draw back your left foot and bring the legs together.

Suggestions for the Concluding Exercises

Each time you lower your hands while exercising, you also lower the blood in circulation. As a result, anyone who has circulatory problems might become dizzy. If this is true for you, do not direct your concentration downwards.

When doing the concluding exercises, women who are menstruating should not place their hands on the lower abdomen (lower *Dan Tian*), but on the middle of the chest (middle *Dan Tian*), so that the collection of blood in the lower body is not forced. It is best if each woman investigates these effects for herself.

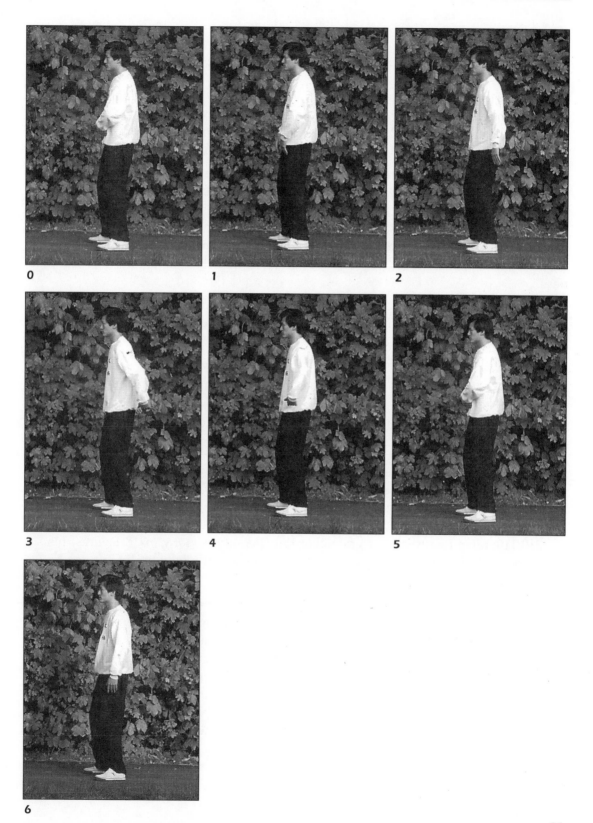

0

1

2

3

4

5

6

◆ QIGONG HARMONY IN 18 FIGURES

Introduction

The original Chinese name for this set of exercises is "Taiji Qigong in 18 Figures." It means Qigong exercises in 18 figures similar to Taijiquan exercises. It was developed by Master Lin Hou Sheng in 1982. The exercise has since become very popular among millions of people in China, South Asia, America, Europe, Japan and Australia.

The 18 Figures are easy to learn, and very effective for maintaining health and curing illnesses. The exercise series promotes overall wellness, and is especially good for the back, kidney and lumbar areas, for bone diseases, the sciatic nerve, obesity, inflammation in the shoulder joints, high blood pressure, heart disease, emphysema, asthma, chronic hepatitis, chronic kidney inflammation, diabetes mellitus (sugar-diabetes), gastro-intestinal inflammations, physical weakness, exhaustion, insomnia, and nervousness.

Regular practice of the 18 Figures usually leads to better health in about a month. The practice of individual figures can also heal certain illnesses.

Healing Successes:

According to the official statistics (1987) of the Institute for Traditional Chinese Medicine (TCM) in Shanghai, one of the most important institutes in China for research of TCM, the following medical cases were positively influenced by Qigong Harmony in 18 Figures.

Example 1: Mr. Chen, 54 years of age (without a declared occupation); Diagnosis: High blood pressure. Was treated without success by both Western medicine, and the Phytotherapy of Traditional Chinese Medicine. The patient suffered from dizziness and a feeling of weakness, and needed a walking cane. Blood pressure 210/110; after two weeks of practicing the Qigong Harmony in 18 Figures, his blood pressure sank to 140/90, remained stable, and the patient did not need a walking cane.

Example 2: Mr. Liu, 45 years of age, teacher; Diagnosis: superficial gastritis, bleeding from a duodenal ulcer and inflammation of the esophagus, four months of black stool. All previous treatments were unsuccessful. The patient had no appetite and showed weight loss; anemia, hemoglobin 9.8 g/dl; patient stopped taking medications, and began to practice Qigong Harmony in 18 Figures. After one month's exercise the stomach pains disappeared, the patient had a good appetite and felt full of energy. Hemoglobin rose to an almost normal level of 12.8 g/dl. After six months of exercise, the recurrent colds of some years were also cured.

Example 3: Mrs. Gu, 40 years of age (without a declared occupation); Diagnosis: Lack of blood platelets and anemia; skin with blue splotches, bleeding at the gums. Special results in blood tests: Thrombocytes 80 000/µl, red blood cells 2.85 Mio/µl, Hemoglobin 7g/dl. Although the patient first felt very weak, after a month's practice of the 18 Figures, she again had energy, could walk, and ride a bicycle without difficulty for a long time; blue splotches on skin and bleeding of the gums disappeared. Blood analysis: Thrombocytes 120 000/µl (strongly improved), red blood corpuscles 4.50 Mio/µl (normal), Hemoglobin 12 g/dl (normal).

Example 4: Mrs. Fu, 38 years of age (without a declared occupation); for two years she had swollen feet with pain, and could not wear shoes. Despite physical examinations in several Hong Kong hospitals, cause of illness could not be determined. After seven sessions of the 18 Figures, the symptoms improved consistently; after ten sessions, the edema in her feet was gone, and the patient could walk normally in shoes.

Example 5: Mrs. Hao, sixty years of age, manager; Diagnosis: lung cancer. Treated surgically in a Peking-hospital, she suffered a relapse and was no longer operable. The patient had no strength and could only go short distances. After two months of practice of the 18 Figures the patient felt better and stronger and could swim; at the same time, the leucocytes (white blood cells) rose from 3700/µl to the normal amount of 7800/µl. For eight years her physical condition has been excellent.

Example 6: Mr. Wu, twenty-six years of age, student; Diagnosis 1978: schizophrenia (Central Psychiatric Hospital in Shanghai). Treated with electro-shock, released after eight months; 1979 relapse. Mr. Wu practiced Figure 2 and Figure 12 with significant improvement of the symptoms; he had an appetite, slept well, remained in a good mood, and the need for medication declined significantly. For eight years his situation has been stable.

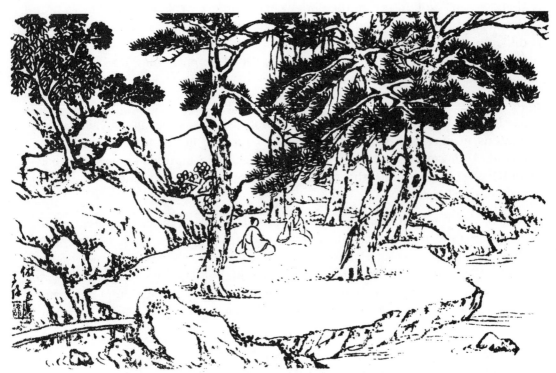

Reproduction of a drawing from the Qing dynasty, circa 1670 A.D.

Description of the 18 Figures

This series is best practiced in the morning after waking up and in the fresh air; in the evening before going to bed; and sometime during the course of the day, for a total of three times. Each figure of this series should be performed six times, unless otherwise indicated, before going on to the next figure. Inhalation and exhalation are counted as one time.

The duration of the exercise with all 18 figures lasts from 15 to 20 minutes, and can be performed for a longer or shorter period, for example, if only individual figures are practiced.

Explanation of the Scale

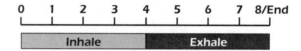

This scale is provided for the benefit of those without access to an instructor or the videotape that accompanies this book. The scale is a simple visual reference for breath coordination and the speed of each movement. Because you will perform the movements at your own speed, this scale does not follow a pre-determined time limit (for example, five seconds for each movement). Instead, you set the pace and apply it to the scale. This is similar to performing a piece of music or a dance—the tempo can be determined by the performer.

The numbers on the scale correspond to the numbers beneath each photograph. In some cases (for example, Figure 3—Moving a Rainbow,) you will return to a photo several times. Simply follow the numbers under the photos in the order they appear on the scale.

Other Notation

- Inhale/Exhale: Denotes inhalation and exhalation.

  The period of inhalation and exhalation can vary in length, that is, measure 1-4 can be counted more quickly or slowly than measure 5-8.

- Previous Figure: Transition from the previous figure.

- Basic Posture: Transition to basic posture which only occurs if no further figure follows.

Figure 1: *Awakening the Qi*

Effect: This exercise awakens the Qi, activates the meridians, regulates the Qi and blood circulation, and sets the rhythm for the entire exercise. It has a quieting effect, especially on high blood pressure, and a healing effect on heart and liver diseases, as well as on insomnia.

Starting Position: Assume a relatively lower standing position, hands beside the body, eyes looking straight ahead and the face relaxed.

When Inhaling: Slowly lift your hands to shoulder height, arms outstretched. Keep your elbows straight and let the movement come mostly from your shoulder joints. Let your hands hang with relaxed wrists. As you inhale, you can straighten your legs, but not so high as to lock the knees. While gradually going up, take care that your upper body is not inadvertently bent forwards or backwards, or that your stomach is pushed forward. When raising your arms, do not hunch your shoulders. Your pelvis should not tilt forward.

When Exhaling: Return to the starting position. Let your hands sink with their palms pointing to the ground; the fingers are also stretched but without effort; go back to the starting position, let your hands fall to your sides and straighten the pelvis. As you do so, do not bend the upper body backwards, but straighten the pelvis without straining the abdominal wall.

Conception: When rising you collect the good Qi. Concentrate on the body. The body relaxes itself in order to let the Qi flow. When exhaling, the body again relaxes, and bad influences are transmitted down through the feet into the earth.

Suggestion: Be sure that your whole body remains relaxed, and let the entire movement take place as harmoniously as possible.

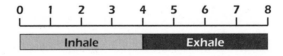

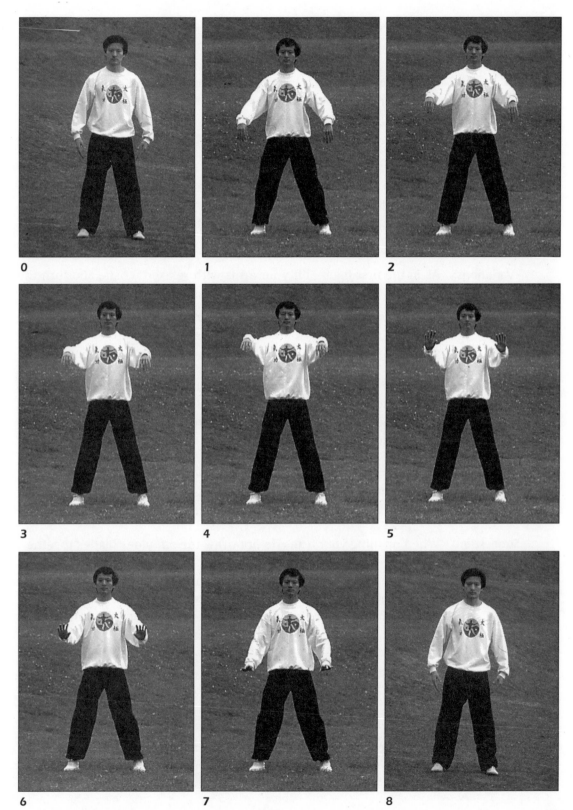

0

1

2

3

4

5

6

7

8

Figure 2: *Opening and Expanding the Chest*

Effect: Removes tensions in the chest, helps against diseases of the lungs, like asthma; helps against heart diseases, heart palpitation, blockages of breathing, feelings of pressure in the chest, and against neuroses and other psychic ailments.

Starting Position: A lower basic position (rider position).

When Inhaling: At the end of the first figure, turn the palms of your hands to face one another, lift the arms again to shoulder height, and then open them completely. At the same time, slowly stand higher, and look straight ahead.

Variations: As in the first figure, lift your arms with relaxed wrists, and turn the palms of your hands to one another at shoulder height.

At the end of the inhalation your legs are straight but not locked, the weight is equally distributed on your feet, and your body's center of gravity is between the legs.

When Exhaling: Close the arms until they are parallel, turn the palms of your hands down, and let the hands and arms sink as in the first figure. At the same time, lower your knees back to the starting point of the standing position.

Conception: Imagine that you are on a beach or mountain top, and there is nothing to disturb your view of a boundless horizon. You breathe freely of the fresh air and feel carefree and happy.

Suggestion: When opening your arms do not draw the shoulder blades together; the space between them should remain open. Keep space in the arm pits, and when opening your arms, imagine that the joints of the shoulders expand and your arms become longer. Also with this movement the shoulders should not be hunched, but remain relaxed.

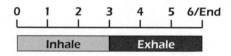

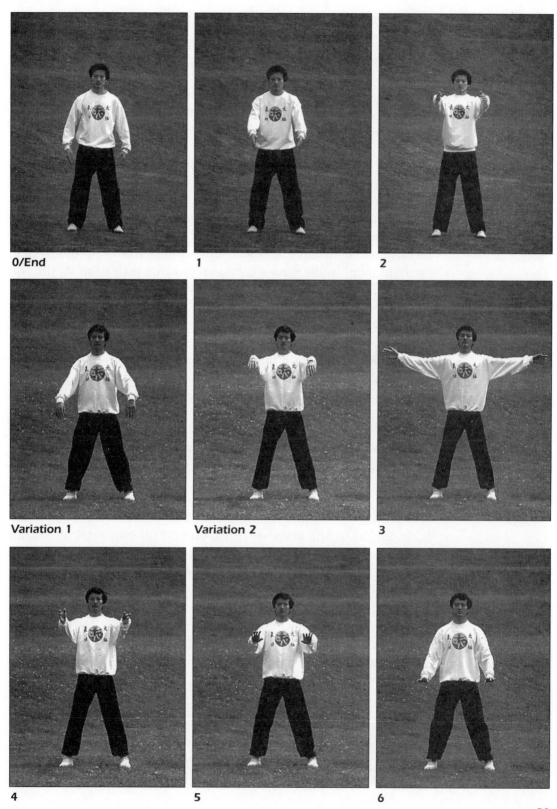

0/End

1

2

Variation 1

Variation 2

3

4

5

6

Figure 3: *Moving a Rainbow*

Effect: Helps relieve lower spine and back pain and makes the waist more slender.

Starting Position: Subsequent to the second figure, you are in the same starting position as in the first figure.

When Inhaling: Gradually lift your hands with relaxed wrists, as in the first figure, to chest height, and then move your left hand to the left side, and lift your right hand above your head. At the same time, put your body weight on the right leg, and let the left leg gradually straighten. At the end of the inhalation, the palm of your left hand should face up and be at shoulder height. Bend your right arm slightly with the palm of the right hand facing somewhat down towards your head. At the end of the inhalation, stand as depicted in the photograph.

When Exhaling: Shift your weight to the left leg. Let your right hand sink to the right, to shoulder height—the palm of the hand now points up. Lift and bend your left arm until the palm of your left hand somewhat faces the top of your head. At the end of the exhalation, stand on the left leg, with the knee bent; your right leg should be straight with no weight on it.

Conception: Imagine a rainbow which you gently swing back and forth with your hands. Cultivate a feeling of inner peace and happiness.

Suggestion: The lifting and sinking of both arms must be flowing and harmonious. Halfway through the weight shift from leg to leg, your whole body, including the arms and legs, should be symmetrical. Do not hunch your shoulders, and do not hold your arms at the same vertical plane. The whole movement should feel natural and pleasant. When inhaling, place the weight on your right side and move your arms to the left. When exhaling, do the reverse. With the last exhalation let your hand drop down instead of to the right. At the end of each inhale and exhale, the side of the body with the unweighted leg should be relaxed.

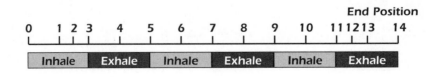

40

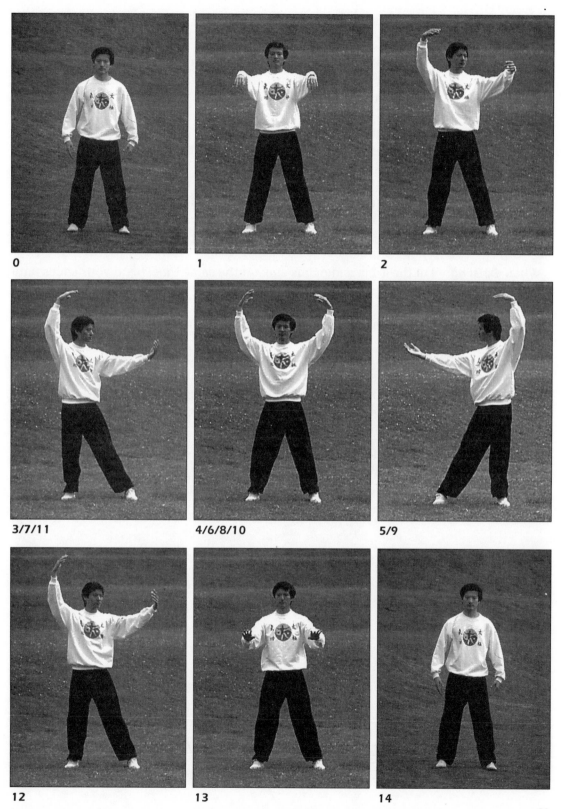

0

1

2

3/7/11

4/6/8/10

5/9

12

13

14

Figure 4: *Pushing the Clouds Apart*

Effect: To collect the original Qi, to strengthen the leg and lumbar muscles. Helps in cases of heart diseases, asthma, and inflammations and ailments of the shoulder joints.

Starting Position: Subsequent to the third figure, stand in the rider position. Let your hands sink to pelvis height and cross at the wrists. The palms of the hands point towards your body.

When Inhaling: Turn the palms of your hands up, and cross them upwards and in front of your body while gradually and gently straightening your legs. When your hands are over your head, turn the palms outward.

When Exhaling: Let the arms and palms sink. At the same time, bend your knees until you are back in the rider position.

Conception: Hover among lovely clouds, part them with your hands, and feel happy.

Suggestion: Your arms should not be stretched with effort, and your shoulders should not be drawn up. When inhaling, you can slowly raise your head to get a deeper breath. When exhaling, let your head gently drop. Your body should feel relaxed.

If you suffer from high blood pressure, do not lift your hands higher than your chest or face, and keep the palms of your hands facing down. When lowering your hands, let them sink sideways from the face or chest.

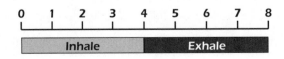

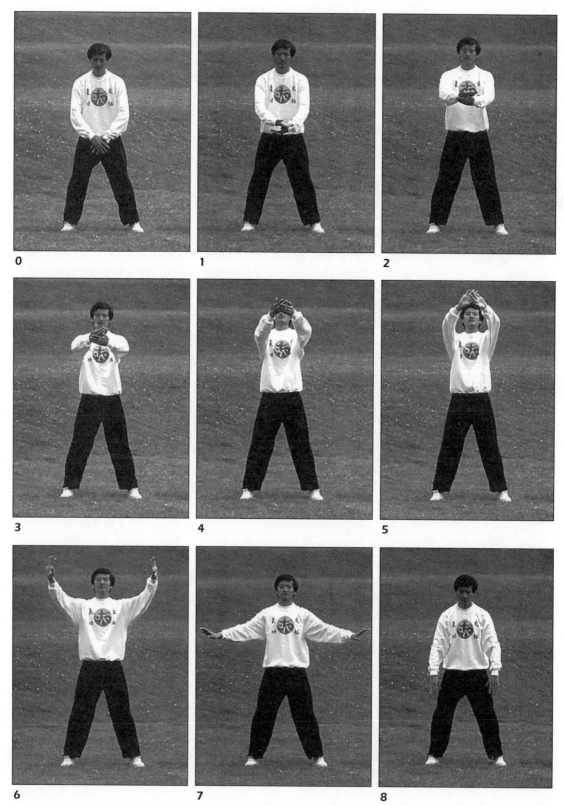

Figure 5: *Rolling the Arms*

Effect: For ailments of the shoulders, elbows, and wrists. Helps against asthma, inflammations of the respiratory tract, and diseases of the kidneys.

Starting Position: Rider position.

When Inhaling I: Stand subsequent to the fourth figure in the rider position with your hands crossed above your head, palms facing up. Let your left hand fall to shoulder height. Bend your right elbow and describe a curve with your hand to approximately ear height. Then turn your shoulders to the right, and look at the right hand. Again push the right hand forward by your ear, and at the same time draw your left hand back to your body. When your hands meet one another, begin to exhale.

When Exhaling I: Push your right hand with an upright palm forward, following it with the eyes, and draw your left hand towards the body. Then turn your shoulders.

When Inhaling II: Turn your shoulders further to the left and direct your eyes to your left hand. At the same time, turn the palm of your right hand upward so that it lies somewhat crosswise, and the left hand somewhat upright. Again, bring the left hand past the ear and follow it with your eyes. At the same time, draw your right hand back.

When Exhaling II: Draw the right hand back to the body and push the upright palm of the left hand forwards.

Direct the movement left and right while breathing in and breathing out.

Conception: Imagine a lovely ocean beach, with the waves rolling forward and back. Move your hands in this rhythm. At the inhale, if the hand that is going backwards describes a curve, imagine that you embrace and breathe in the best Qi. When exhaling, both hands pass each other, and you imagine that your hands touch the surface of an inflated balloon.

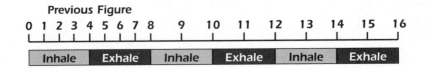

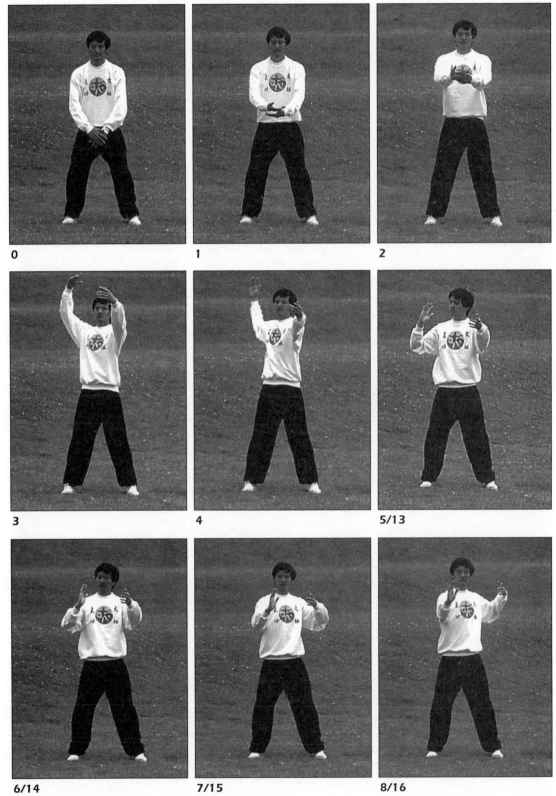

0

1

2

3

4

5/13

6/14

7/15

8/16

Suggestion: Pushing the hands forward and drawing them backward happens when the body is relaxed; that is, you let an inner force move your hands. Your eyes should always follow the hand that is going forward.

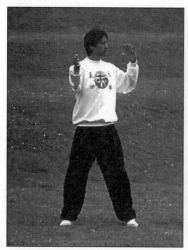

9

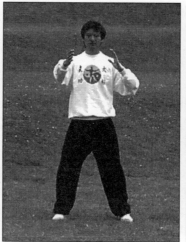

10

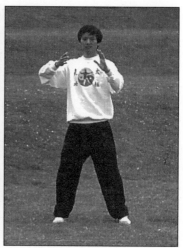

11

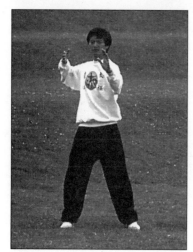

12

Figure 6: *Rowing on a Calm Lake*

Effect:	Strengthens the digestive system; helps prevent heart disease and inflammation of the gastro-intestinal tract; strengthens the nerves. This figure is especially refreshing, and good for clearing the head. As an independent exercise, you can repeat it as often as you like.
Starting Position:	Subsequent to the fifth figure at the exhalation your hands meet, and you turn your palms down and let your hands, as in the first figure, sink sideward along the body and behind it. At the same time, bend your knees, keep your upper body straight, and keep your eyes forward. Press the palms of your hands backwards as far as you can. Exhale during the entire movement.

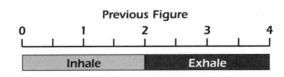

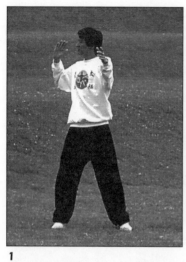

1

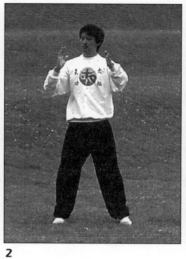

2

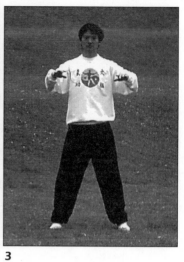

3

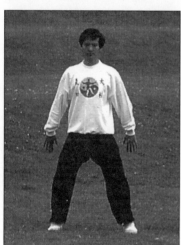

4

When Inhaling: Stand a little higher, stretch the arms, and make a circular movement upwards, outward, and to the sides. The palms of your hands should point forward at the end.

When Exhaling: Bend the knees again, let your hands sink, and guide them as far as possible backward.

Conception: Peace, composure, freedom. Imagine that you are rowing over a calm lake, enjoying nature.

Suggestion: When exhaling, keep your arms straight and relaxed. They should not be stretched with effort. Consciously drop your shoulders. When inhaling, slowly stand higher; when exhaling, lower. Do not bend your upper body too far forward or backward.

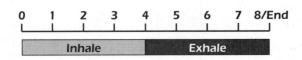

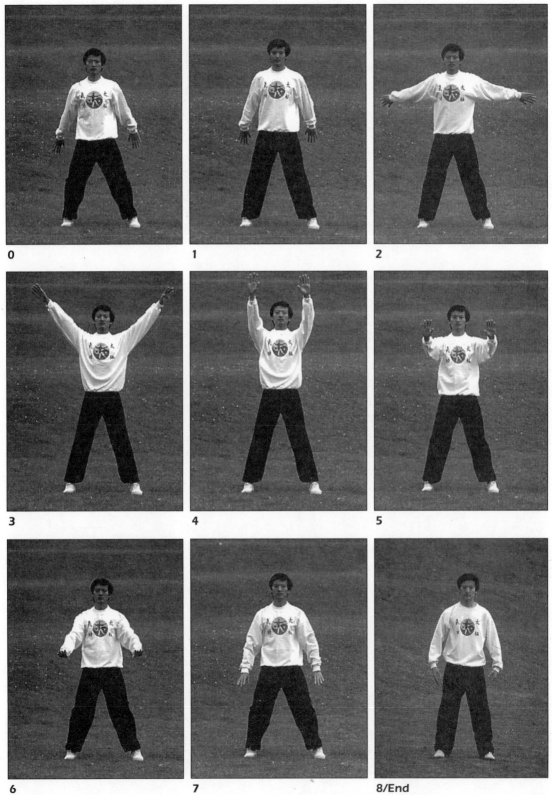

0

1

2

3

4

5

6

7

8/End

Figure 7: *Lifting the Sun with a Hand*

Effect: Promotes relaxation of the chest and deeper breathing. Helps soothe physical and mental stress and illness.

Starting Position: Subsequent to the sixth figure, let your hands again sink back to their basic position.

When Inhaling: Turn the palm of your right hand diagonally to the left, and put your body weight on the left leg. Stretch both legs slowly, lift your right hand forward to shoulder height, and hold the palm of your hand upwards. While keeping your weight on the left leg, raise the heel of your right foot, keeping the tips of the toes on the ground. Look into the distance.

When Exhaling: Return to the starting position.

Inhale again, and repeat the movements on the opposite side: lift your left hand, shift the weight to the right leg, and then return again to the starting position when exhaling.

Conception: Feel like a happy child playing with a ball. Look far into the distance, and lift the sun over the horizon. From your arms to your hands you can feel a connection with the sun.

Suggestion: When raising your hand, look out over your hand and then into the distant horizon. When raising your hand, leave the point of the unweighted leg on the ground. Your breathing should be harmonious.

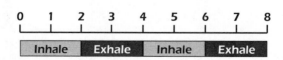

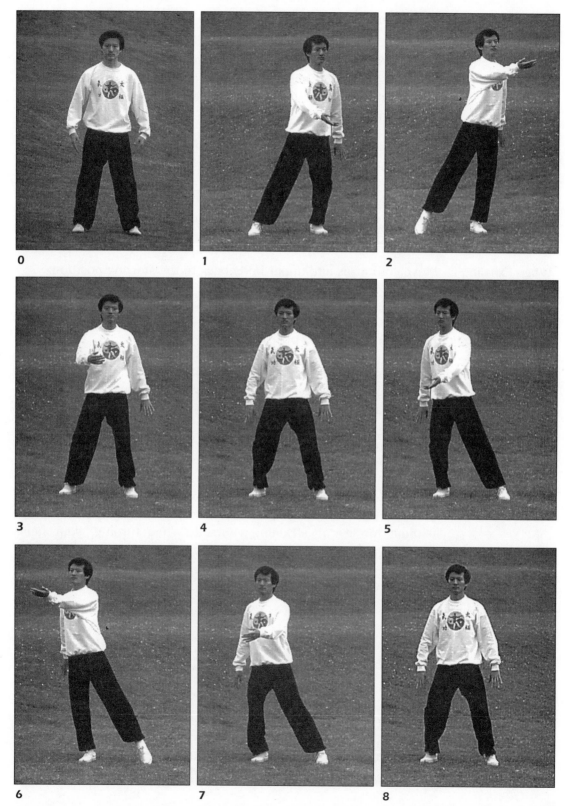

0

1

2

3

4

5

6

7

8

Figure 8: *Turn the Head and Look at the Moon*

Effect: Strengthens the spleen and kidney system, is effective against back pain and discomfort and weakness in the lumbar muscles, and good for weight regulation. This exercise can also be performed independently, and as often as desired.

Starting Position: Subsequent to the seventh figure, starting from the "rider" position (basic position).

When Inhaling I: Lift and lightly stretch your arms behind and to the left of your torso, turn the upper body, and direct your gaze up along your raised hands as if you were looking at the moon.

When Exhaling I: Move your arms and upper body back to the starting position.

When Inhaling II: Perform the same movements to the right.

When Exhaling II: Return to the starting position.

Conception: On the 15th of September, the eighth month in the lunar calendar, the Chinese celebrate the full moon with a moon festival. The round full moon is also a symbol of completeness. All members of the family gather to celebrate, and the family is united and happy. With this conception, you should turn your gaze to the moon to feel sheltered and happy among family and friends.

Suggestion: Raising the hands and turning the upper body and head should take place harmoniously and synchronically. Turn as far back as you can without forcing or straining yourself. When turning, your heels should remain on the ground.

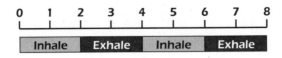

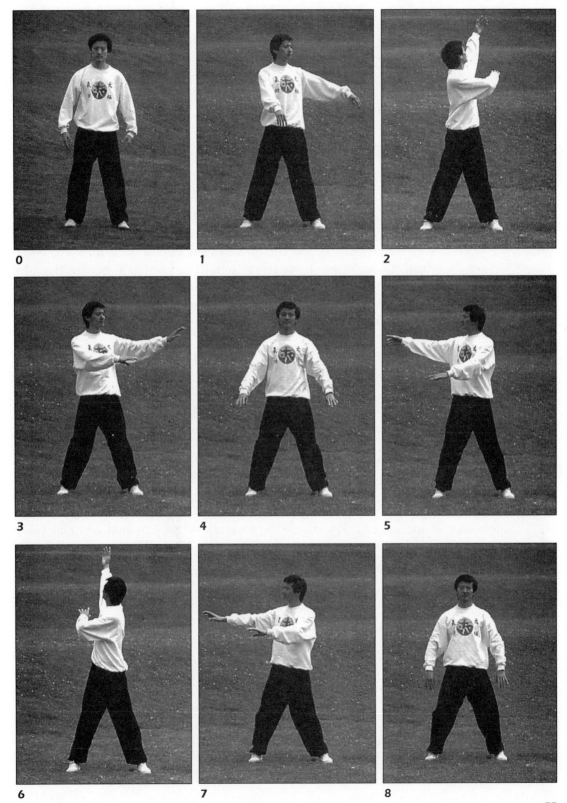

0

1

2

3

4

5

6

7

8

Figure 9: *Turn the Upper Body, Push the Palms of the Hands*

Effect: Strengthens the lumbar muscles and spleen-kidney system. Improves the mobility of the upper body and of the upper extremities; has a healing effect on back ailments, the lower spinal column, and the legs.

Starting Position: Subsequent to the eighth figure you stand in the "rider" position, with your hands at your waist; the palms of your hands face up, and you inhale.

When Exhaling I: Turn the upper body to the left, and with inner force move the right hand diagonally to the left. The palms of your hands thus remain somewhat vertical, and the edges of the hands point forward. When turning your upper body to the left, draw the left shoulder, the connecting arm, and the hand to the rear for counterbalance.

When Inhaling I: Move your shoulders, arms, and hands back to the starting position.

When Exhaling II: Repeat the movement on the other side; thus your left hand moves to the right, and the upper body to the right and behind, and so forth.

When Inhaling II: Return to the starting position.

Conception: Concentrate on breathing in the good Qi, replenishing and strengthening your inner power. Relax the entire body, and preserve inner peace.

Suggestion: Your whole body should be relaxed. When exhaling you can place your weight on the left side when you push the hand, but it is not necessary.

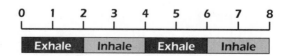

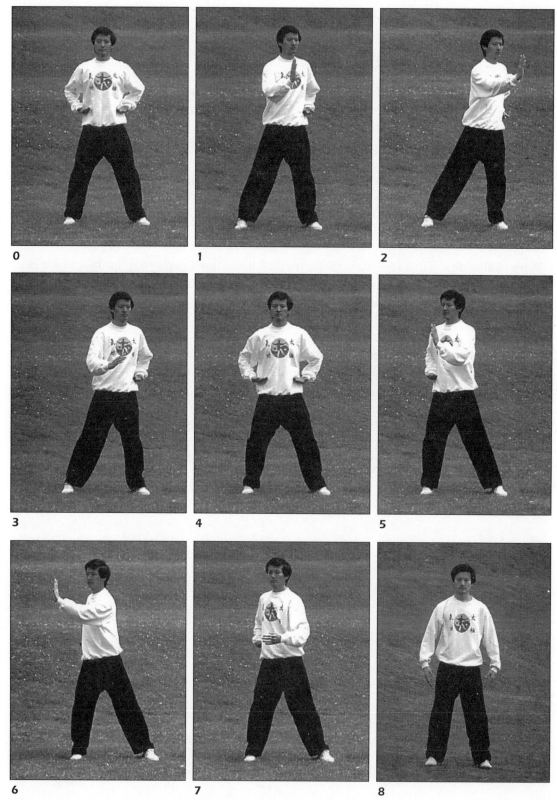

0

1

2

3

4

5

6

7

8

Figure 10: *Hands of the Clouds in Riding Position*

Effect: Helps against weakness of nerves, neuroses, and gastro-intestinal illness, e.g. bad digestion. Promotes refreshment of the body and improvement of the memory. This figure is recommended as an independent exercise because of its distinct revitalizing effect.

Starting Position: Subsequent to the ninth figure.

When Inhaling: Turn the palm of your left hand toward your body, stretch your right hand forward to the height of your navel. Hold the palm of your right hand so that it faces to the left, and then turn the upper body to the left.

When Exhaling: Turn the palm of your right hand inward to your body and lift it to the height of your eyes. Let the left hand drop to navel height, and let the palm of your hand point to the right. Then turn your upper body to the right side.

Conception: Sense how your hands, arms, cervical vertebrae, and head are united. Your arms, torso, and legs should move harmoniously with each other.

Suggestion: Your hand motions should be gentle and your body should not be stiff or tense. Direct your gaze to the upper hand, which is moved by your body.

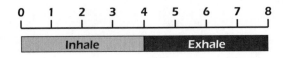

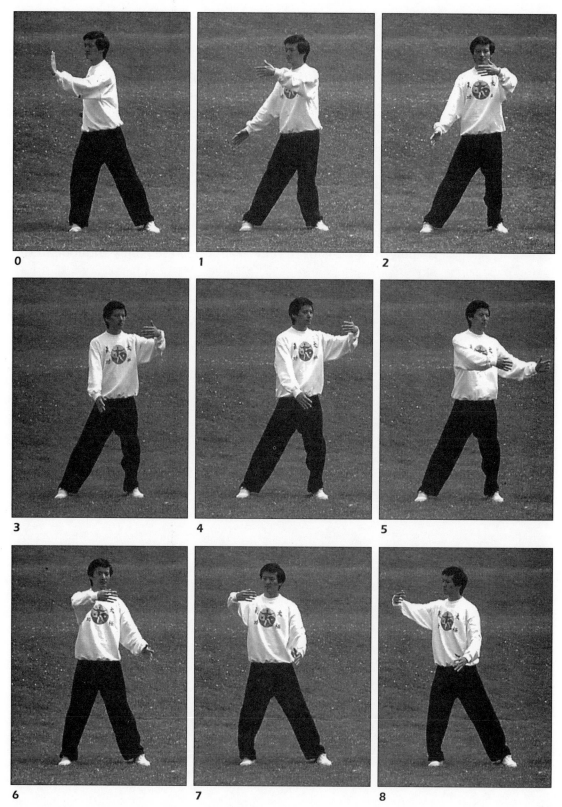

0

1

2

3

4

5

6

7

8

Figure 11: *Grab the Bottom of the Sea, Look to the Sky*

Effect: Fortifies the kidney and spleen systems, strengthens the lumbar and leg muscles, and helps against illnesses of the gastro-intestinal tract. This figure is effective against ailments and difficulties in moving the lumbar area and legs, and contributes to weight regulation.

Starting Position: Subsequent to the tenth figure. With your left foot take a curving step (Gong Bu) forward, bend your body forward and bring the arms down until the wrists cross in front of the left knee. Exhale during the entire movement.

When Inhaling: Gradually straighten your upper body and bend backwards, while holding your arms over your head. Open the palms and look to the sky.

When Exhaling: Begin to exhale with your arms spread out. Turn the palms of your hands face down, bend the body forward again and guide the arms down in front of the left knee.

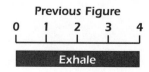

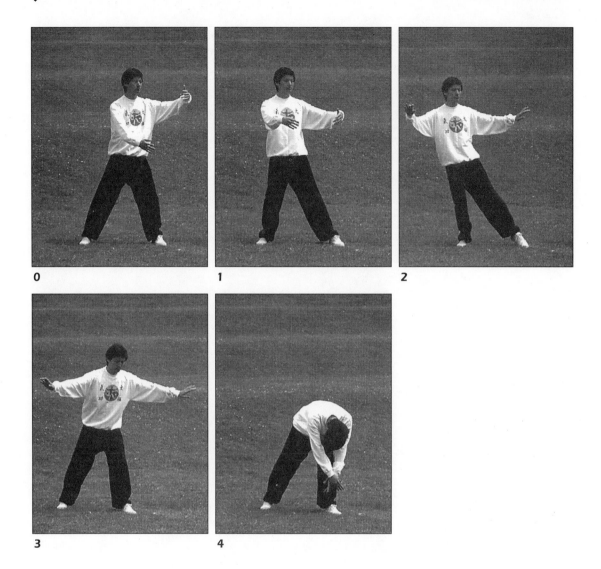

0

1

2

3

4

Conception: Reach into the depths of the sea and scoop up water. Your glance to the sky and the opening of your arms should give you a joyful, liberating feeling.

Suggestion: Lift the arms parallel over your head, and then begin to straighten the upper body, so that the leverage effect is intensified. When your body is bent backwards and the arm movement ends, the arms are straight. This figure can be performed as often as you wish, as both an independent exercise, and with a change of the leg positions.

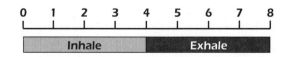

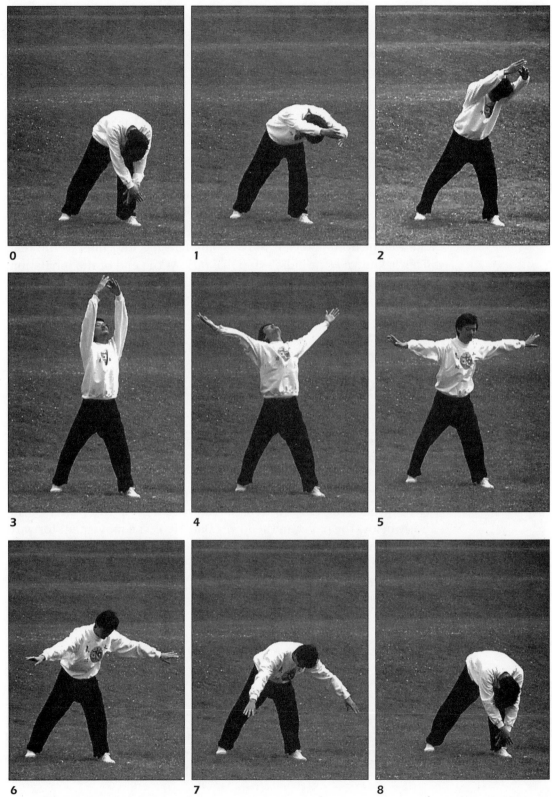

Figure 12: *Move the Waves*

Effect:	Strengthens the liver and spleen systems and has a healing effect on hepatitis, illnesses of the lungs, nerve pains between the ribs, neurasthenia and insomnia.
Starting Position:	Subsequent to the eleventh figure. Your left foot is forward and your right foot is back.
When Inhaling:	Raise your arms to about chest height; at the same time, raise the upper body slowly and draw in the elbows until your hands are in front of your body at about chest height. At the end of the inhalation the palms of your hands face forward. When moving your body, shift the weight from your left leg to your right leg, and thus to the rear. This is known as an "idle" step *(Xü Bu)*. At the end of the inhalation, stand almost completely on your right leg, with the right knee bent. Your left leg should be straight and unburdened and resting only on the heel.
When Exhaling:	In one movement, move the upper body and the palms of your hands forward. The tips of your fingers should be at about eye height. Shift your body weight gradually from your right leg to your left leg until a left curving step is made.
Conception:	Move a great sea wave forwards and backwards, or let your body be moved by the waves.
Suggestion:	Shift your body weight backwards when inhaling, and simultaneously draw back the elbows. The movement starts in the center of the body below the navel, in the lower Dan Tian. The movement forward should come from the Dan Tian and torso, not the hands. The body, arms and hands accompany the movement of the palms. When shifting the weight forward, you can go beyond the curving step, so that your heel is raised. The twelfth figure should be repeated twelve times.

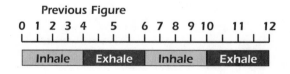

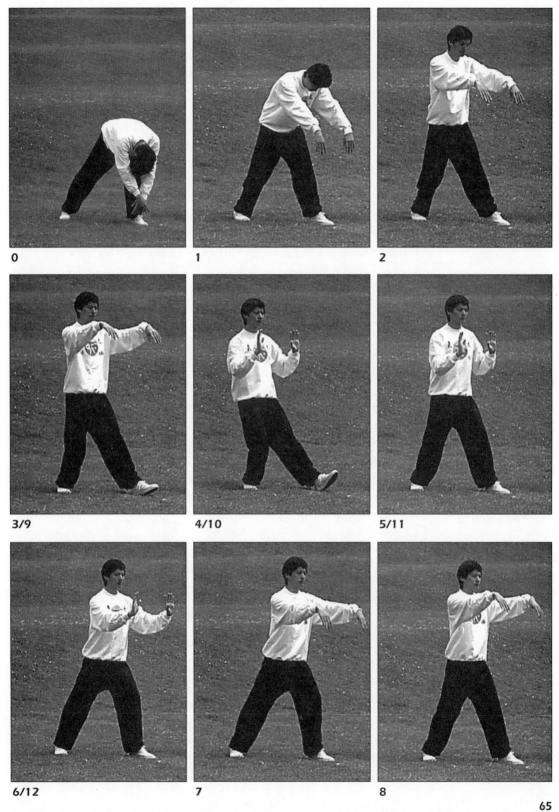

0

1

2

3/9

4/10

5/11

6/12

7

8

Figure 13: *The Flying Dove Spreads Its Wings*

Effect: Has an harmonious effect on the liver and spleen systems; helps cure hepatitis and lung diseases, pressure in the chest, heart disease, and neurasthenia.

Starting Position: Continuing on after the twelfth figure, turn, with nearly straight arms, the palms of your hands towards one another at the end of the exhalation. Your left foot is forward, and the right foot backward.

When Inhaling: Open your arms until they are spread out. At the same time, shift your body weight to the right leg. At the end of the inhalation only your right leg is weighted; your left leg is empty, the ball of the foot is lifted, and only your heel touches the ground ("idle" step).

When Exhaling: Close your arms again with the palms facing each other, and shift your weight forward onto your left foot ("curving step"), as in the twelfth figure.

Conception: Rise easily and naturally, like a dove, into the blue sky. Fly with a feeling of happiness, breathe in fresh air, and enjoy nature.

Suggestion: When shifting your weight forward, you can go beyond the curving step so that your right foot no longer completely rests on the ground and the heel is raised. When spreading your arms, imagine how a dove opens its wings; feel that you are flying backwards. When closing your arms you should be completely relaxed, just like a bird. Repeat twelve times. This figure can also be practiced independently with a change of the foot position.

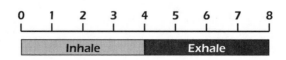

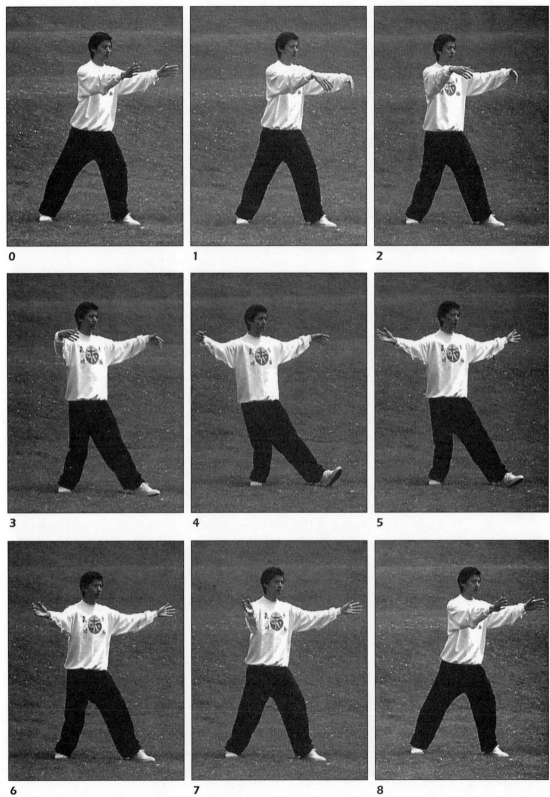

0

1

2

3

4

5

6

7

8

Figure 14: *Push the Fist and Stretch the Arm*

Effect:	Promotes the original Qi, strengthens and harmonizes the body. Increases lung capacity; helps cure asthma, bronchitis, neurasthenia, neuroses, and insomnia. Strengthens the leg muscles.
Starting Position:	Subsequent to the thirteenth position, assume the rider position, and hold your fists next to your waist (see photo 0). The backs of the fists points down; thumbs point outward, and the elbows are drawn back. Inhale in this position.
When Exhaling I:	Push the left fist straight ahead and at the same time turn your shoulders to the right (the right shoulder moves back). Follow the moving fist with your eyes.
When Inhaling I:	Return to the starting position.
When Exhaling II:	Push your right fist forward and turn your shoulders to the left (the left shoulder moves back). Follow the fist with your eyes.
When Inhaling II:	Return to the starting position.
Conception:	This figure comes from the Chinese art of self-defense. Move your body as a single unit, and use your inner strength to push a great weight with your fist while turning your upper body.
Suggestion:	The rider position is a deep standing posture. Your feet should be parallel, and about shoulder-width apart. You should feel as if you are riding on a horse. The fists make half a turn when going forward so that the back of the fist faces up. The fist is then approximately at shoulder height. If your legs get tired, you can stand higher in order to prolong the duration of the exercise.

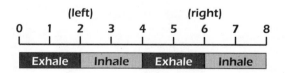

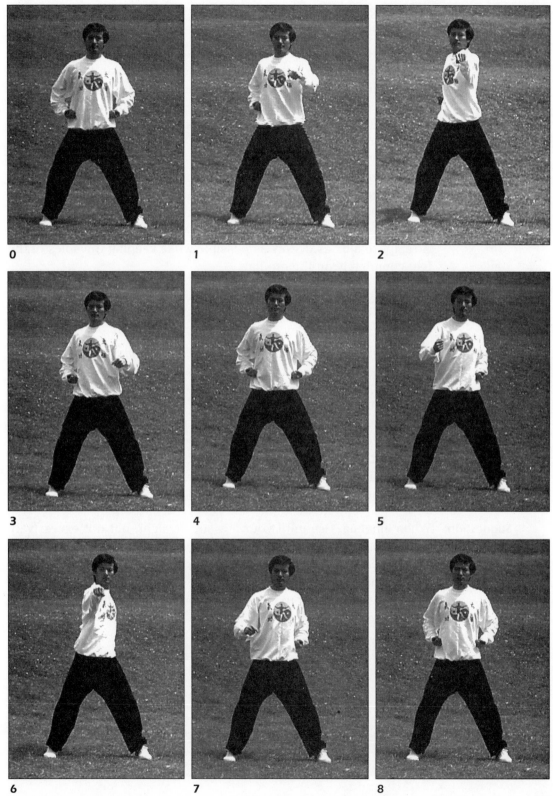

0

1

2

3

4

5

6

7

8

Figure 15: *Fly Like an Eagle (or a Wild Goose)*

Effect: Relieves inner tension, works against nervousness, feelings of dizziness, neurasthenia, neuroses, and the feeling that the head will burst. When practiced alone, this figure is good for all chronic illnesses, since it harmonizes the body, relieves inner tensions, and has a liberating effect on the body and spirit. Its effect is based mainly on its inner calmness and feelings of joy and freedom.

Starting Position: Subsequent to the last exhalation and drawing back the fist in Figure 14, gradually stand a bit higher. When exhaling, bend your knees more deeply while keeping your upper body straight. Open your fists, and let your hands sink down along the sides of your body. Attempt to sink as deeply as possible while keeping the soles of the feet completely on the ground.

When Inhaling: Slowly rise up, and lift your arms with palms of your hands facing down.

When Exhaling: Sink down while your arms remain horizontal; only the wrists drop a little.

Conception: In China this figure is named after the wild goose. This bird is the embodiment of freedom. With it comes spring, and thus it is the herald of a lovely season. When inhaling you rise, like an eagle or wild goose, into the sky. When exhaling, float freely again to the earth. Feel free and happy, and experience the wide, open sky and the vastness of the world.

Suggestion: When inhaling, rise until your legs are straight, but not excessively stretched. If you have good stability, you can lift yourself onto the balls of your feet. This reinforces the feeling of rising and flying. When exhaling, first settle back onto your heels and then sink down. Your wrists ought not to be cramped, but should follow your breathing and body movements.

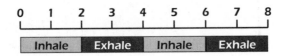

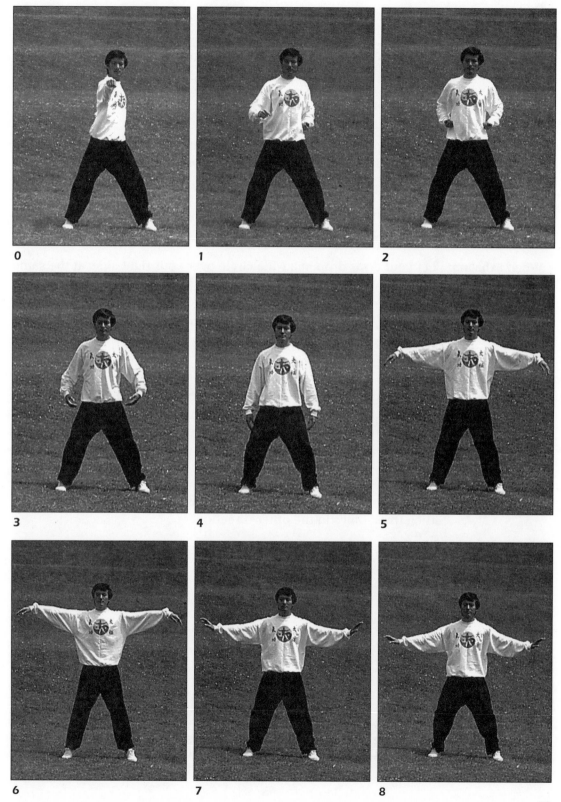

Figure 16: *Revolve Like a Windmill*

Effect: Promotes circulation of the Qi and blood, refreshes and harmonizes the body, strengthens the spirit, and awakens joy for life. Helps against arthritis and other ailments of the joints, and also helps to keep one trim.

Starting Position: Subsequent to the previous figure, return with the last exhalation to the starting position, and bend the upper body forward.

When Inhaling: Lift your arms in a broad circle over your left side until they are above your head. Make a corresponding circular movement with the pelvis over the right side and forwards.

When Exhaling: Let your arms drop in a wide circle over your right side; at the same time, move your pelvis from the forward position to the left and back.

Conception: The whole body turns like a great windmill in a gentle breeze at sunrise. The turning embraces the cosmos; nature and the body become one.

Suggestion: The movement of arms, pelvis, and breath should be harmonious. The exercise is easier if you bend your upper body less. Discover for yourself how far to bend without discomfort. You can repeat the exercise more often and more slowly so that no feeling of dizziness occurs. If you feel dizzy, rest for a moment before continuing.

The exercise should be repeated three times in one direction, and then three times in the other direction.

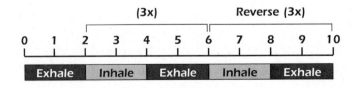

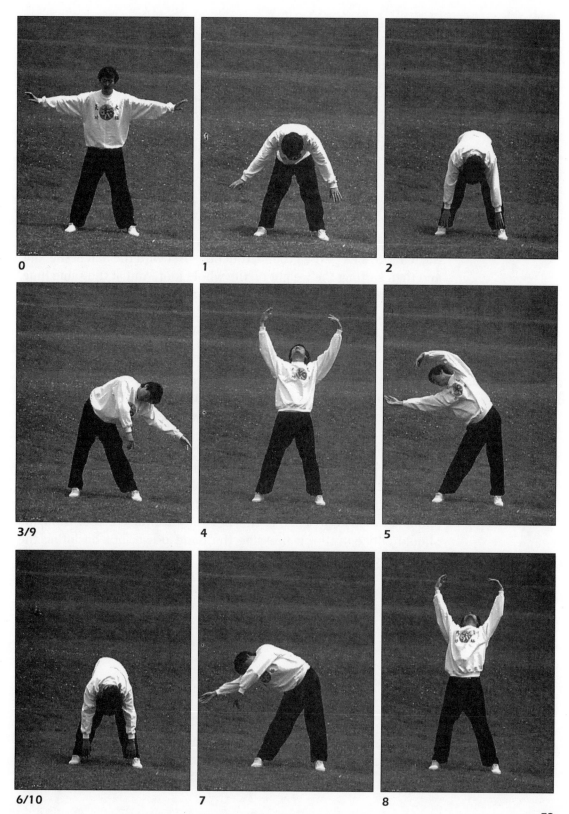

0

1

2

3/9

4

5

6/10

7

8

Figure 17: *Play with a Ball Like a Child*

Effect:	Effective for tired muscles, lack of strength, and spiritual and bodily exhaustion. Helps against neurasthenia and stiffness in the hands and feet. Harmonizes the body movement, and brings about a feeling of cheerfulness, and helps also with feelings of melancholy. This exercise is especially recommended for older and weaker persons.
Starting Position:	Subsequent to Figure 16 you straighten up. Bring up the left knee, and raise your right hand to shoulder height. You are now in the starting position.
When Inhaling:	Press the palm of your right hand down next to your upper thigh; let the left foot sink to the ground, touching first with the ball of the foot, and then settling the weight on the whole foot. And at the same time, raise your left hand to shoulder height and raise your right knee.
When Exhaling:	Press the palm of your left hand down and let the right foot sink to the ground. Then raise your right hand and your left knee.
Conception:	Feel carefree and happy like a child, and imagine you are walking in a beautiful environment with lovely flowers and fresh air. Admire nature at sunrise while playing calmly with a ball.
Suggestion:	Stand upright and keep your upper body and pelvis straight. Raising and lowering your hands and feet should be synchronous with your breathing. The whole body should be relaxed, especially in the area of the kidneys and lower spinal column. Your feet and their joints should always be relaxed, even when they are raised. Your thoughts should concentrate on pressing the hand down, not on lifting the other hand.

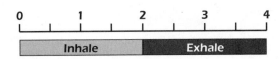

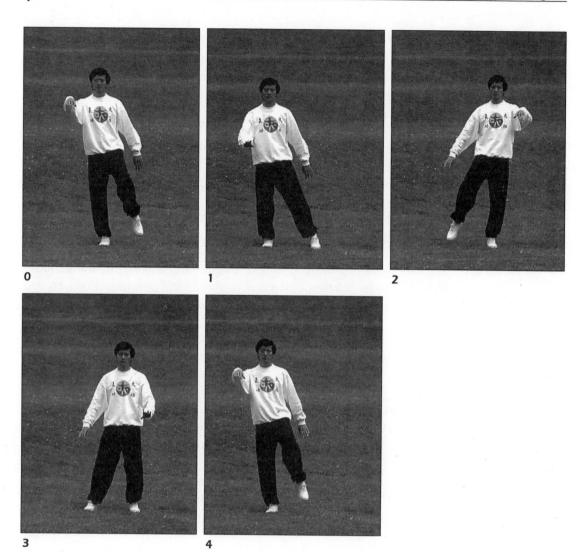

0

1

2

3

4

Figure 18: *Quieting the Qi*

Effect: Produces inner peace and calmness; works against high blood pressure and disturbances of the cardiovascular system and the gastrointestinal tract.

Starting Position: In the starting position you stand upright. Place your hands in front of the lower body, with the palms of your hands facing up, and the fingers approximately pointing to one another.

When Inhaling: Lift your hands to about eye level and at the same time stand slightly higher, palms facing your body.

Variations: Starting from the basic position, inhale and move your hands sideward to the front and upwards with the palms pointing down, to eye level. At the same time, slowly raise your body higher.

When Exhaling: Turn the palms of your hands down, always with the finger tips pointing towards one another; press your hands down and, at the same time, bend your knees slightly.

Conception: The heart beats quietly and the Qi flows in harmony with your breathing and body movements. Create an internal and external readiness to end the exercises, and gradually conclude.

Suggestion: Through practice and observation, find out for yourself how high your hands need to be raised and where exactly the palms of your hands should point so that you feel good when exercising, and do not mistakenly direct the Qi to one side more than the other and feel unwell.

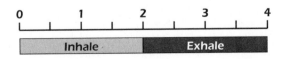

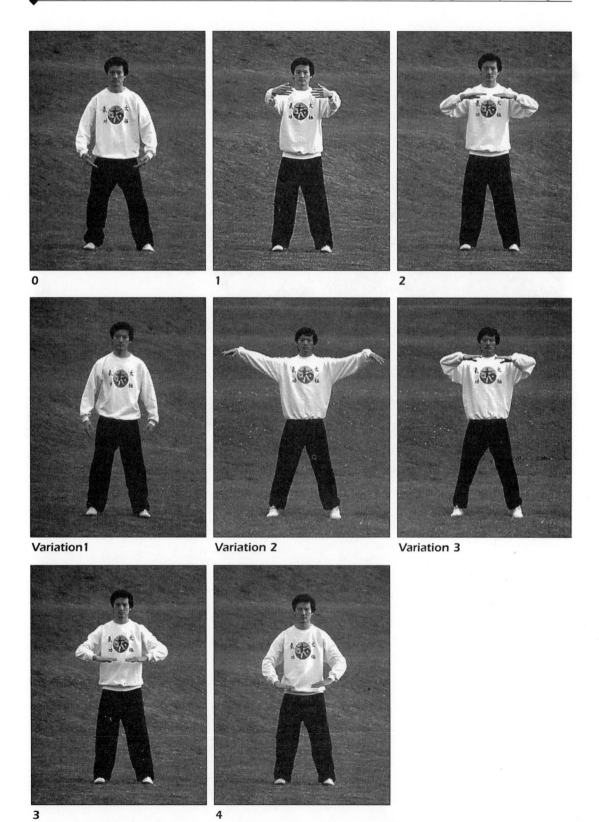

0

1

2

Variation1

Variation 2

Variation 3

3

4

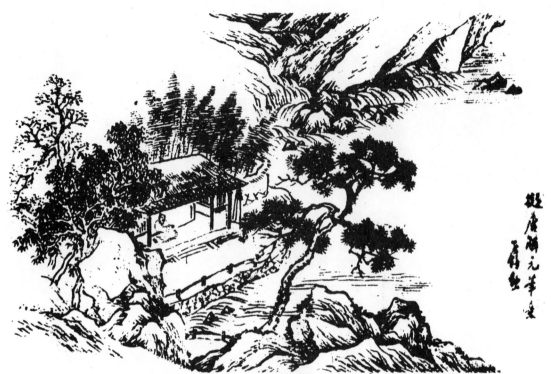

Reproduction of a drawing from the Qing dynasty, circa 1670 A.D.

◆ The Eight Figures for Every Day

Introduction

The Eight Figures are very well known in China. Almost all employees and students in the cities practice these figures every day. Daily at 10 A.M. and at 4 P.M., the Chinese central broadcasting station sends out an announcement (with accompanying music) of the Eight Figures.

I remember well the time that I studied medicine in Beijing. At 10 A.M. every day a long break was taken. Almost everywhere I saw students practicing the Eight Figures for Every Day. It lasted about a quarter of an hour, and was a very pleasant change in student activity. At the same time a break was taken in factories and businesses, giving everyone a chance to practice this sequence.

The movements of these figures were developed from classical Chinese health exercises, and partly from the art of self-defense (exercises for body and mind).

The goal is to train your body every day. If you want to do something for your health, you will find in these Eight Figures exercises that are suitable to activate meridians and joints, to stretch the tendons and sinews, and to train the muscles. These exercises are especially appropriate if you cannot regularly find much time for sport. With five to ten minutes daily, you can improve your health and prevent "getting rusty" from a lack of movement.

These exercises are not only effective on the physical body. Through their specific movements, they affect the flow of Qi. These exercises are also appropriate for warming up for other Qigong exercises.

You can perform them slowly and meditatively, or with music. If practiced in a group to music, then follow the beat of a Viennese waltz. Count for all figures from 1 to 8. For the seventh figure count more slowly, and in the eighth figure count double-time.

From 1 to 4 the practice begins on the left side, from 5 to 8 on the right side. Each figure is usually practiced four times; that is, do the first figure four times, then the second figure four times and so on. If you have more time and inclination, you can repeat all the figures, or spend a longer time with each figure. For regular practice it is wise to maintain the sequence of the exercise, since this activates the body, and thus the Qi, in a gradual, sensible manner, and unites the different figures in a harmonious fashion. Finally, you can practice each figure as often as you like and need.

DESCRIPTION OF THE 8 FIGURES

Figure 1: *Movement of the Upper Extremities*

Movement 1: move your left foot a step to the side so that your feet are approximately shoulder-width apart, and the weight evenly distributed. At the same time, turn the palms of your hands out, reach up and out with the arms, close the hands into fists, and draw them downwards to the shoulder-joints.

Movement 3: keep your hands closed into fists, and again extend your arms until they are parallel, and then turn your face upwards.

Movement 6: bring your fists in front of your shoulders and look forward. Angle your wrists so that the fists turn inward, then turn your fists and wrists forward and to the outside, and extend your arms horizontally.

Movement 7: close your legs and let your arms sink beside the body and open your hands.

Movements 8 to 14: reverse the beginning movement so that your first step is with the right foot instead of the left. Then continue the exercise as listed above.

All eight movements of this figure are easy to learn, and have great benefits. This first figure moves all the upper extremities, from the shoulder-blades and head to the shoulder-joints and finger tips, so that all possibilities of movement are played out. In the first piece, you turn the palms of your hands outward, and thus move the arms in their shoulder joints. Making a fist involves movement of the finger joints, and pulling down moves the joints of the elbows. In the second piece, the shoulders are raised, and the elbows stretched. In the third piece, the wrists move with the angling and turning of the fists. In the fourth piece, you return to the starting position, and all your extremities relax. The complete figure expands and stretches the body in the same way you do naturally when yawning.

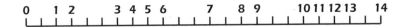

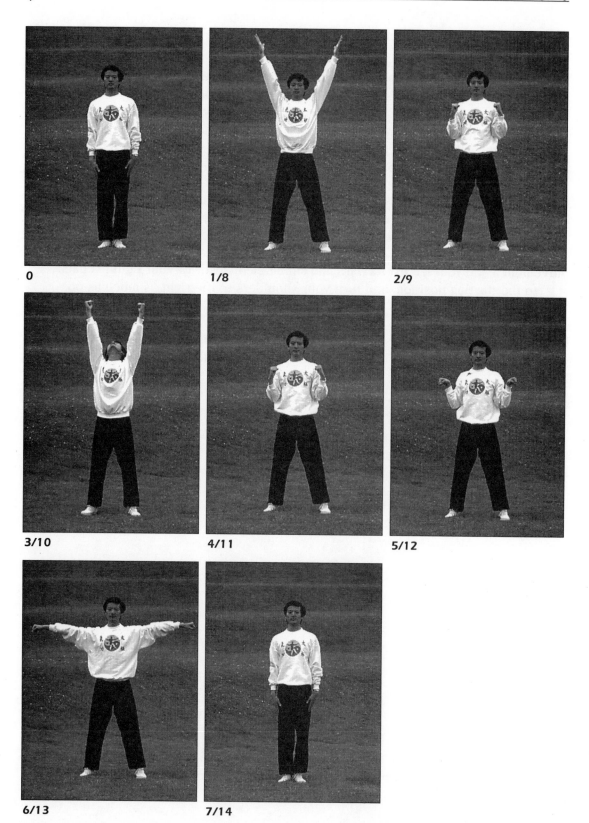

0

1/8

2/9

3/10

4/11

5/12

6/13

7/14

Figure 2: *Movement of the Fist Jab*

Movements 0 through 3: make a fist of your right hand and hold it at hip level. Move your left foot in a curving fashion to the left side, and at the same time move your left hand in an arc in front of your body. The left-hand palm is upright with the fingertips pointing up. At the end of the arc withdraw the arm, gradually making a fist with the thumb on the outside. At the end both fists are beside your hips, and your feet are parallel and pointing diagonally to the left.

Movement 4: the right fists jabs forward, and the shoulders turn as much as possible to the left. The fist does a half turn when going forward, so that the back of the fist faces up at the end of the movement.

Movement 5: jab your left fist forward and simultaneously draw your right fist back to the starting position, and turn your shoulders to the right as much as possible.

Movement 7: draw the left fist back to move to the starting position—feet together, both fists beside the hips, elbows drawn backwards, and eyes front.

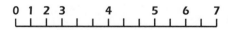

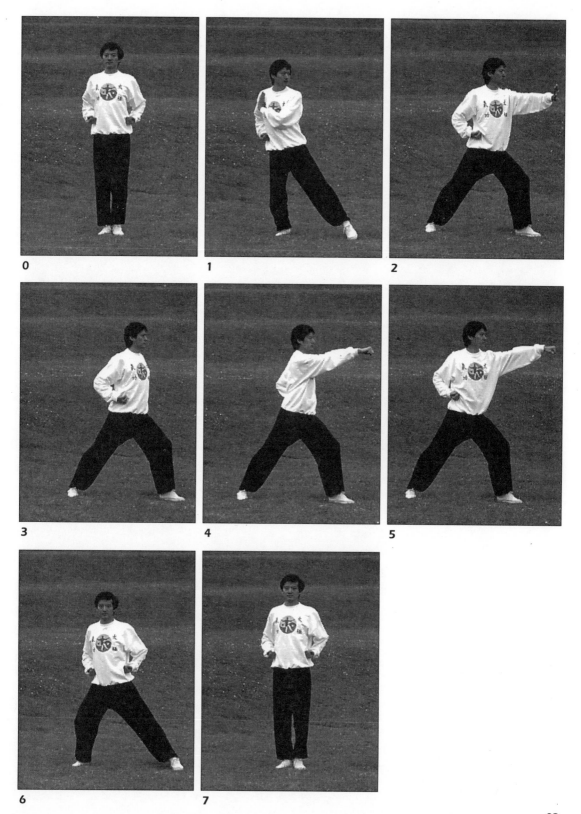

Movements 7 through 14 are the reverse of movements 0 through 6. Make the beginning step with your right foot instead of your left, move the right hand in a circle and in 11 the left fist jabs forward.

7 8 9 10   11   12   13   14

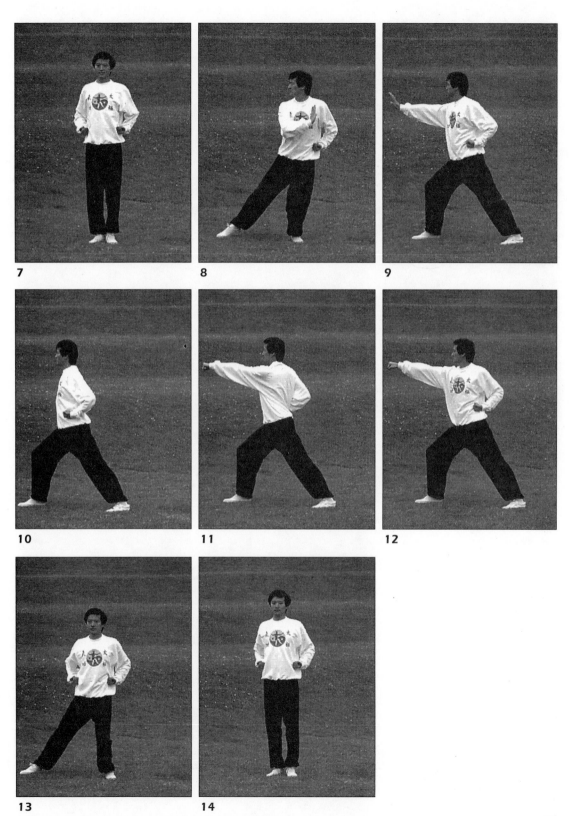

7

8

9

10

11

12

13

14

Figure 3: *Expanding the Chest*

Movements 0 through 2: move your left foot forward in a curve step fashion; at the same time, extend both arms forward and then to the sides, so that the chest and inner sides of your arms are stretched. Make your hands into fists.

Movements 3 and 4: once again bring your arms together and then open them to stretch the chest.

Movement 5: step back with your left foot, then put both hands on your knees. Bend your knees as far as possible while keeping the heels of your feet on the ground and your back straight.

Movement 6: stand up again.

Movements 7 through 12 repeat on the other side so that the curving step is done with your right foot.

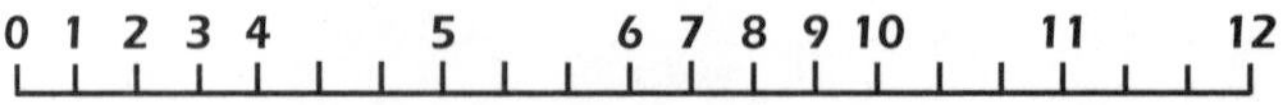

```
0 1 2 3 4      5      6 7 8 9 10      11      12
```

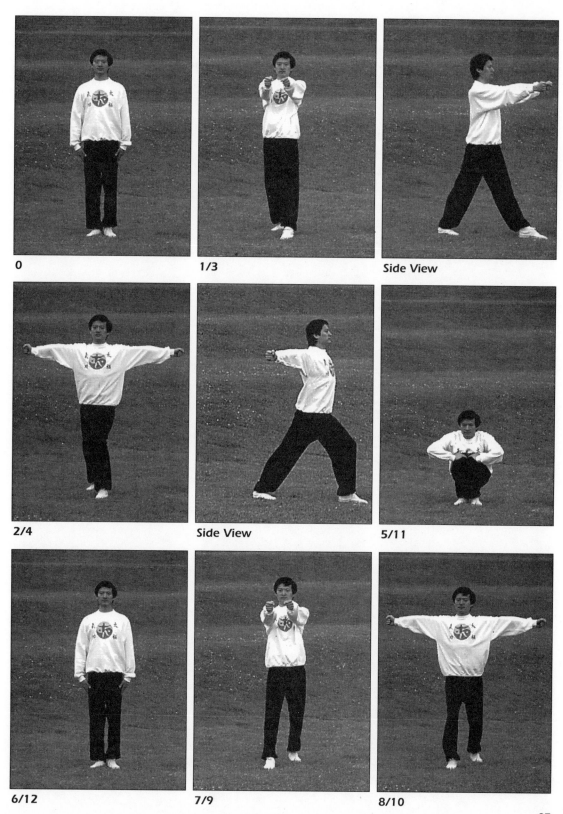

0

1/3

Side View

2/4

Side View

5/11

6/12

7/9

8/10

Figure 4: *Swinging the Legs*

Movement 1: take half a step forward with your left foot and put your body weight on your left leg; at the same time, open both arms to an angle of 60 to 90 degrees.

Movement 2: swing your right leg out in front of the body. Keep the legs straight, and if possible touch the upper part of your foot with both hands. Keep your back straight and do not lean forward to try and touch your foot.

Movement 3: same as movement 1.

Movement 4: return to the starting position and bring the arms to the sides of the body.

Movement 5 to 8 are not pictured. Simply reverse the pattern so that you step forward with your right leg and swing your left leg.

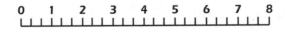

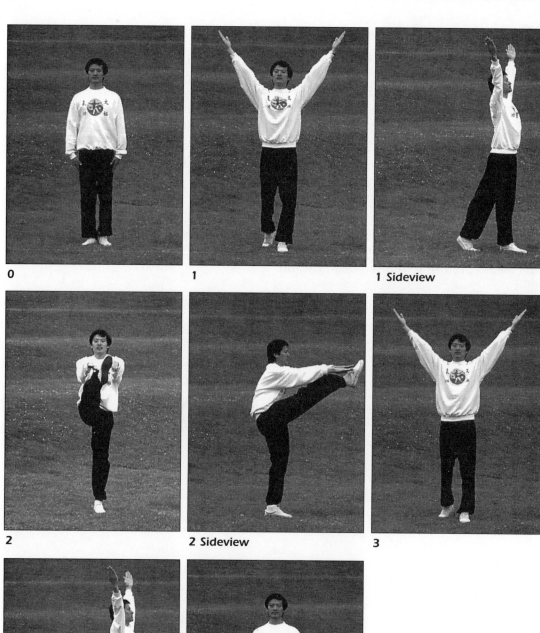

0

1

1 Sideview

2

2 Sideview

3

3 Sideview

4

Figure 5: *Bending the Upper Body*

Movements 1 and 2: step far out to your left side with your left foot so that your feet are parallel and your toes point forward. At the same time, lift your left arm in a circular motion sideward until it points directly up. Place your right hand on your right hip. Then, in a continuous motion, bend the upper body to the right so that you feel a stretch in the left side of your body and the inside of your right leg. Your body weight is now mainly on the left leg, and your left knee is bent; your right leg is tense like a bow string, and your whole upper body inclines to the right.

Movements 3 through 6: repeat the bending and stretching of the body.

Movement 7: return to the starting position.

Movements 8 through 14 are again reversed so that your right foot steps out to the side.

```
0  1  2  3  4  5  6    7  8  9 1011 1213   14
└──┴──┴──┴──┴──┴──┴────┴──┴──┴──┴──┴──┴──┴──┘
```

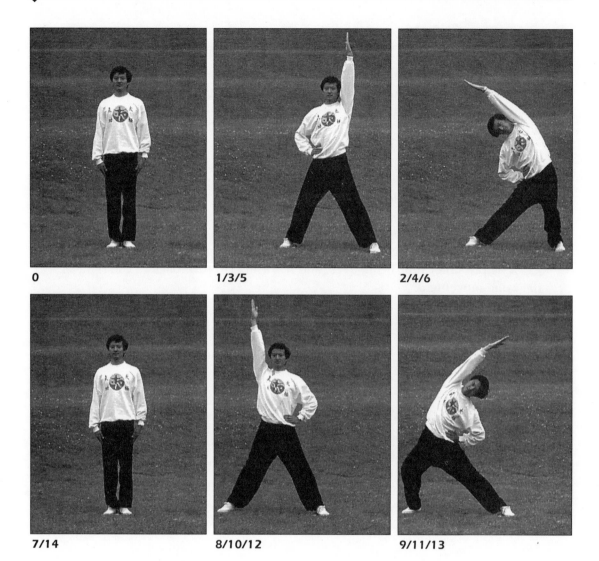

0

1/3/5

2/4/6

7/14

8/10/12

9/11/13

Figure 6: *Turning the Upper Body*

Movement 1: take a half step to the left so that your feet are about shoulder-width apart with your body weight distributed evenly between your legs. At the same time lift your arms horizontally to shoulder height with the palms facing down.

Movement 2: bend your upper body to the left and down until your right hand reaches the tip of the left foot. At the same time the left hand goes up as if both arms were fixed to a pole.

Movement 3: straighten up again, make your hands into fists and turn your upper body back and to the right, raising your right arm diagonally back to the right as far as possible. Your head, eyes, and left arm also turn back to the right in the same movement.

Movement 4: return to the starting position.

Movements 5 through 8: reverse the sides and perform the same movements.

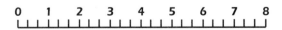

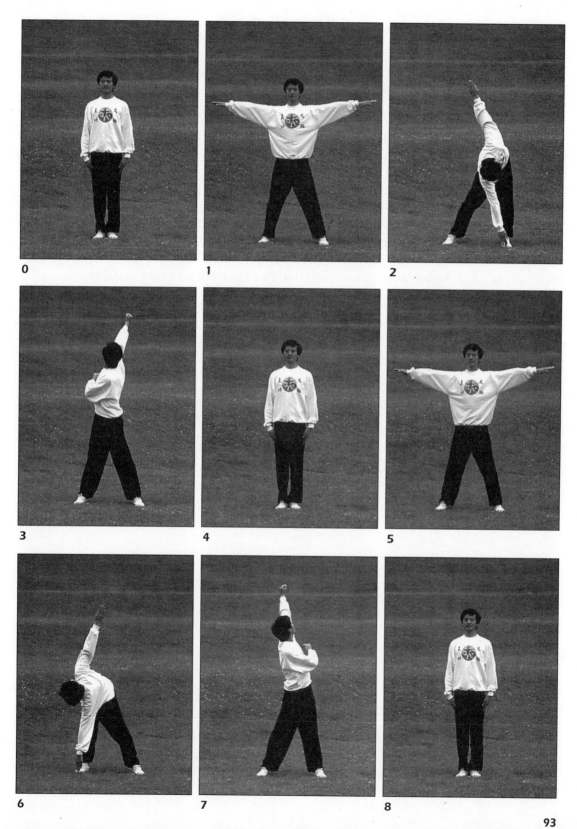

0

1

2

3

4

5

6

7

8

Figure 7: *Train the Stomach and Back Muscles*

Movement 1: raise your arms above your body so that the palms of your hands face forward, and bend the upper body backwards.

Movement 2: bend your upper body, keeping the legs straight, and attempt to touch the ground with your fingers.

Movement 3: straighten your body and open your arms above your head at an angle of 60 to 90 degrees, with the palms of the hands turned towards one another. At the same time, make a forward curving step with your left foot.

Movement 4: return to the starting position.

Movements 5 through 8 are in reverse, so that in 7 the right foot makes the forward curving step.

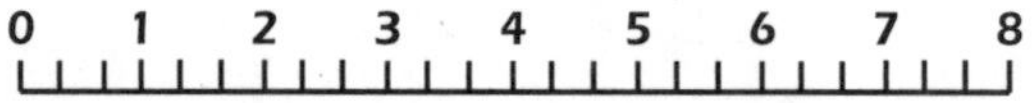

0   1   2   3   4   5   6   7   8

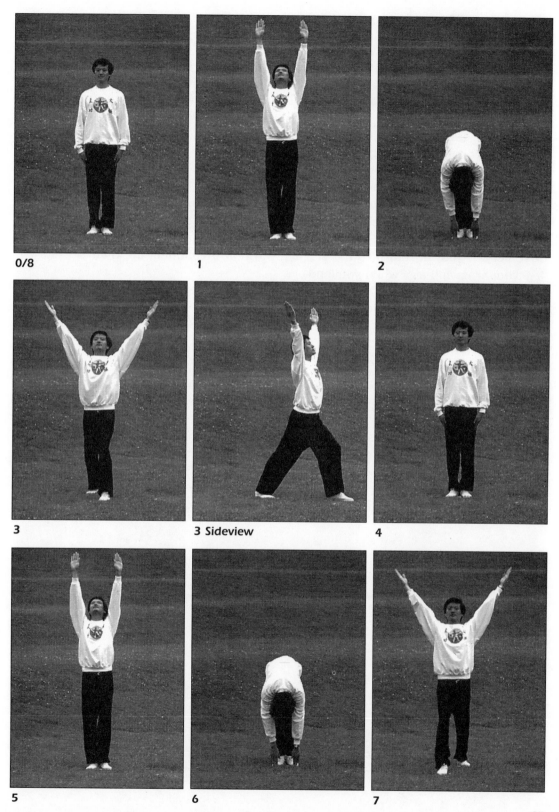

0/8

1

2

3

3 Sideview

4

5

6

7

Figure 8: *Jumping Exercise*

Movements 1 and 2: jump up and open your legs so that your feet are parallel and approximately shoulder width apart; at the same time stretch out your arms horizontally, with the palms of your hands facing down. Keep your arms out when you land.

Movements 3 and 4: jump again. Close your legs and clap your hands above your head. Keep your hands together when you land.

Movements 5 and 6: return to movement 1 by jumping up, opening your legs, and dropping your arms to shoulder height, palms facing the ground.

Movements 7 and 8: return to the starting position by jumping up, then closing your arms and legs when you land.

Movements 9 to 16 are a repetition of the same sequence.

0 1 2 3 4 5 6 7 8 9 10 11 12 13 14 15 16

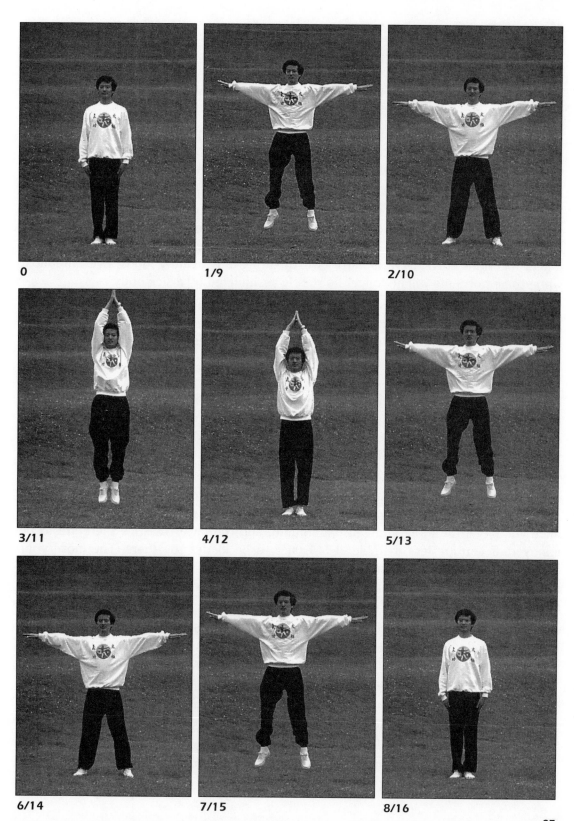

0

1/9

2/10

3/11

4/12

5/13

6/14

7/15

8/16

C) SUGGESTIONS FOR A HEALTHY LIFE STYLE

Some say: "I live well because I don't eat meat," or "I no longer eat sugar and salt," or "I'm dieting." It is true that the kinds of foods you eat play an important role in health. However, many people remain healthy even if they do not observe the rules of nutrition, while others, despite diet and precautions, get ill.

Cows eat hay, and produce milk which has many important ingredients for your health. And why? According to some "theories of health" the cows must, of course, first drink milk in order to produce milk. Thus, not only what you ingest plays a role, but also how the body utilizes it.

The body naturally knows exactly what it needs or does not need, in order to be in good condition. Even if the food is not as "healthy" as it should be, the body can choose and absorb important nutrients and eliminate the unnecessary. But, if the body no longer functions correctly, it is hardly worth eating only healthy foods. Even the most wholesome nutrients will no longer be rightly assimilated by a sick body.

The lesson is that you should not live a "one-sided" healthy life, but a completely healthy life. For example; eat what you want, but not too much and not just that food. The art of healthy living consists of finding the golden mean and living in harmony, so that the body and the spirit function smoothly.

According to TCM you should never overdo anything, even if it is fun or necessary for life. For example, you should not eat too much, dress too warmly, sleep too much, or have too much sex. Moreover, you should limit psychological stresses such as worry, anxiety, sadness, annoyance, and even joy. Avoid desires, entanglements, bad thoughts, and hatred. Excessively loud speaking and laughing are as harmful as unbridled curiosity.

For example, annoyance damages the liver system. How can you avoid annoyance? By showing understanding, being generous, and developing a philosophy that teaches acceptance and forgiveness rather than punishment. The more knowledge and experience you have, the more you can understand, and the fewer reasons there are to be annoyed. If you are less irritable, it is easier to be kinder to others. The more your appearance is positive, such as an open, friendly face, the more other people will respond positively to you. Thus, some irritations that you would otherwise have to combat do not even occur, and your liver is spared!

By means of Qigong exercises you can learn about yourself, in order to find your own needs and limits, and no longer do that which is in fashion, or what some magazine recommends according to current research. These "theories" could be out of date tomorrow.

On the contrary, a healthy life style according to the principles of Qigong is based on the observation of bodily reactions and has proven to be true over thousands of years. As long as the human body does not change, human beings can learn and understand Qigong and use it for further development and discoveries.

You should frequently comb your hair; rub your face; move your eyes; rub over the ears; lick the gums; knock the teeth, collect the saliva and swallow it in small portions;

breath out "sorrowful" Qi, keep your back warm, protect the chest; massage the stomach; tighten the anus muscles; move the joints as far as possible; rub the soles of the feet; dry wet skin completely; wash and massage the body; keep your mouth closed, and do not speak too much.

Once you have learned some Qigong exercises, you should live according to the Qigong principles. For example, just by drawing the shoulder blades apart in a relaxed manner, and keeping the arm pits free, you can remove tensions and pains in the back. In this way, you are continually practicing Qigong. Pay attention when telephoning or typing whether you are inclined to stretch your stomach, or draw up your shoulders. If so, relax your posture. When driving, check your breathing now and then to determine if you are anxious or agitated. Breathe calmly, and thus you can avoid accidents since you will not become nervous or aggressive while driving.

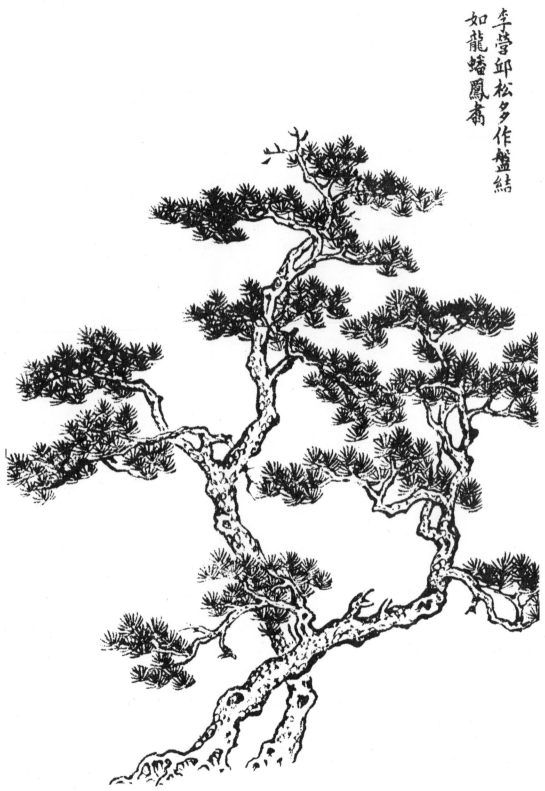

李鱓邱松多作盤結
如龍蟠鳳舂

Reproduction of a drawing from the Qing dynasty, circa 1670 A.D.

CHAPTER 4

Qigong
Questions About the Practice

◆ How do I manage to think about nothing while exercising?

It is very often said in Qigong instruction: "Concentrate on yourself, and think about nothing." That is easier said than done. Precisely when you want to think about nothing, you think of a thousand things. However, to think about nothing does not mean that you shouldn't think about something. Quite the contrary; in order to think about nothing, first direct your attention to something specific. When you concentrate on a specific object, you cannot think about other things. In Chinese it is said: "With one thought, drive away ten thousand other thoughts" (*Yi Nian Dai Wan Nian*).

In Qigong there are different methods of focusing on one thought (which sometimes also help against insomnia). For example, in a state of complete concentration, count from one to a thousand. Another method is to observe your breathing. Try to make your breathing calm and regular. Gradually you become calmer, and at some point, you have gone so far that you no longer think about anything.

In my opinion, the best method is to concentrate on the body. That means observe the body, improve its posture, and relax it step by step. With increasing concentration you turn away from thousands of thoughts, and with the increasing relaxation that results, fewer thoughts assail you.

Investigations prove that even in a half-conscious or hypnotized state, imagining that you have just lifted a bucket results in the tensing of the corresponding muscular system. Even thinking about a movement increases the muscle-tone; and conscious relaxation of the muscles reduces thinking about the corresponding movements. If you think about a tense situation in which you were involved, you are also physically tense. If you are occupied with observation and relaxation of the body, these tense thoughts do not appear. If your concentration leads to an intense relaxation of the body, thoughts no longer have a focus, and you attain a wholly relaxed mood. However, it is important not be so relaxed that you fall asleep when doing a Qigong exercise. Be awake and focused.

Should I exercise with my eyes open or closed?

If you are a beginner, it is recommended that you exercise with your eyes closed so that you are not distracted, and can concentrate better on the body and exercise more deeply.

In time you can keep your eyes open without disturbing your concentration. This is like looking for a key in a purse. You reach in and touch, for example, a handkerchief, button, or coin, and then you find the key. Your eyes are open, but your concentration is wholly on the interior of the purse. It is good if you can transfer this example to exercise.

Concentration works like the caretaker of a house with a flashlight who illuminates every corner of the house in order to check that everything is okay. You want to be aware of every joint and every muscle in order to see if they are in the right condition and relaxed. If this has your attention, you have no awareness of what is outside of you, and thus, there is no disturbance.

If you want to practice with partly closed eyes, begin with your eyes open, and try to direct your vision slowly inward. If you are no longer aware of what is external, the eye-lids partially close of themselves, leaving about 1/3 of the eye open. Do not close your eye-lids tightly—that lends to tension. Concentration directs itself wholly inward during the exercise. But your eyes should be directed straight ahead, not turned upwards.

◆ How does deep breathing take place?

We breathe without use of force. According to the knowledge of Western Medicine, breathing is governed by diverse mechanisms. It is important to know that the body itself regulates the process of breathing.

It is a mistake, in order to breathe deeply, to rapidly and forcefully take in air through the open mouth. The body stops the process suddenly although you feel that there is still room in the chest, and that the lungs are not yet fully expanded.

If you would like to breathe deeply, you must learn to signal to the body that it should breathe deeply. You cannot make "deep" breath. In other words, conscious deep breathing means only letting the body breathe deeply, going along with it, and keeping the chest relaxed.

You can support deep breathing by keeping the respiratory duct (nose) slightly contracted (a little like snoring) when inhaling, and not allow too much air to enter at once. If the supply of air is slowed through some resistance, the chest can expand, and the lungs take in more air. When exhaling, you should also allow the air to escape slowly because the respiratory duct is a bit contracted. Your chest, however, should not be strained.

While inhaling and exhaling, the stream of air should be as regular as possible. Inhalation is generally an energizing process and exhaling a relaxing process. Therefore, you should, when exhaling, be especially conscious of relief. Long and deep breaths help to expand the chest when inhaling, and to achieve relaxation for the whole body when exhaling. The use of power when breathing requires energy, causes excitement, disturbs the regularity of natural breathing, and can even produce pounding of the heart and nervousness. Thus, rigorous and forceful breathing results in tension, and creates the need for more oxygen.

The technique of breathing is nothing more than making yourself conscious of the process of breathing. It is, therefore, not always the same as a specific kind of breathing, such as "stomach breathing" or "deep breathing."

◆ Why should men and women do some exercises from different sides?

According to the principle of Yin and Yang, men represent Yang and women Yin; the left side is Yang, the right is Yin. Therefore, for example, when men do the concluding exercise, they put their left hand on the abdominal wall, and women the right hand. This is also important for the replenishment and dispersion of the Qi.

The principle of Yin and Yang is not a theoretical invention, but a centuries-old physical experience to which you should subscribe. With a long enough experience of Qigong you can determine for yourself what is appropriate and satisfying.

◆ What should I do if my legs tremble or my knees hurt during the standing exercise?

In the correct posture, and if you do not take too deep a stance, your legs should not tremble even if you are not very strong. The feet are parallel in this posture, and the knees are pointing outward, as if you are sitting on a horse. Tension arises which creates a stable position. Should the legs tremble, however, you must correct the posture and internal tension. This is primarily a matter of training.

If your legs are so untrained that they even shake in the correct position, then stand somewhat higher. However, do not stand so high that your knees are completely straight.

Another way to avoid trembling is simply to bend the knees more. In any case, it is a matter of practice and of experience. The correct posture is more important than strength. Thus, these exercises are appropriate for older and weaker people. Through these exercises your legs will be strengthened, and the circulatory system can be stimulated by the flow of Qi.

Pain in the knees may indicate that the knees have not been warmed up before exercise, and are, on the whole, too unfit. If you have problems when climbing stairs, this indicates a lack of Qi in the knee area (through lack of training). In this case, first exercise more carefully and gently and stop if it hurts. Exercise regularly, gradually increase the tension and in time, your knees will become capable of bearing a burden and the Qi flow will improve. A good method against knee pains is to stretch and relax the bend of the knee a few times by touching the toes, as in many of the exercises shown.

◆ Can I by means of expanding the chest area relax tensions there?

No. By experience of the body, tensions or oppressive feelings in the chest area do not come from the chest alone, but arise in connection with other organ systems in other parts of the body.

Chinese Medicine traces these feelings back to a loss or disturbance of Qi, which is brought about by negative influences. You do not do away with these negative influences by expanding the chest, but by supplying positive influences, by naturally deep chest and stomach breathing, and by means of Qigong exercise. You become relaxed and direct Qi through the body, and thus into troubled areas. With general physical relaxation, you become more aware of the existing tensions, and can more easily direct positive influences to them. By means of deep breathing (see above) during Qigong exercise, the chest cavity can be opened and expanded, which can dissolve tensions. If the tension does not disappear immediately, it is certain that it will gradually disappear with further exercise and especially with sensible living.

The question is: how do such tensions come about? They have many physical and psychological causes as has already been explained. Sexuality plays a great role among them. Too much ejaculation leads to loss of the Qi, and to damage of the kidney system which initially causes tensions and pains in the shoulders and back, and then leads to the functional disturbance of other organs. Finally, it comes to organic changes, for example, infirmities of the vertebra, inter vertebral disks, or lumbar muscles.

◆ What can I do against shoulder blade pains?

First, learn the standing exercise correctly. It allows for keeping open or "allowing room" for the armpits. The shoulders drop and relax and the shoulder blades move apart. This posture is part of almost all the exercises, and guarantees the free flow of Qi in the shoulder areas. This alone is already good for tensions in the shoulder blades.

Moreover, you should keep this posture in mind at all times during the day; for example, when riding the subway, standing in line, working, pushing a cart in the super-market, when telephoning and reading, speaking and eating, etc., so that it is constantly in your consciousness, and so that the Qi is not blocked up and pain does not develop.

◆ What should I do if too much saliva collects during exercise?

Exercise produces a saliva flow, and that is a good sign. In classical Qigong teaching, this flow is called *Yu Ye* which literally means "Jade Flow." In China, jade is a valuable object, and is also a symbol for the important kidney system, so the increased flow of saliva is regarded as especially valuable. During Qigong, body fluids, for example, gastric juices, and some hormones are secreted in greater quantity. They are a traceable sign of the Qi flow.

You should swallow the saliva, not all at once, but in small portions, usually in three portions, and then observe where it flows. This procedure creates a Qi flow down to the Lower *Dan Tian* where you usually direct and collect the Qi. Consciously directing the Qi to the Lower *Dan Tian* creates a relaxation of the body as it flows down, relaxes the inner organs, and improves their functionality.

◆ Why do I yawn during Qigong? Does it make me tired?

The influences of Qi are not only transmitted inwardly, but also outwardly. A yawn is an outward transmission. Someone else who is relaxed receives these influences, and yawning can be infectious.

In China, yawning is considered a process of relaxation. Yawning begins physiologically with inhalation, a wide opening of the mouth, and with a corresponding tensing of the muscular system. Relaxation then occurs with involuntary exhalation. Tears sometimes appear in the eyes, and you may get goose pimples. Finally, you feel better and refreshed. This is a result of the flow of Qi. First, the Qi is blocked up in the body, and this creates tiredness. As a normal reaction to this condition the body tenses with yawning, and then relaxes. The blocked up Qi flows through the body, and one feels invigorated.

If you yawn often during Qigong it does not mean that you are tired. During Qigong the body is more relaxed than other times, and thus, more sensitive. It can feel even a small blockage of Qi, and seeks to remove the blockage.

In this way, Qigong can be an effective treatment for insomnia. Anyone who suffers from insomnia usually cannot yawn properly, for the body is not in a position to react correctly to tiredness, although blocked Qi normally creates this reaction. A vicious circle thus begins: lack of sleep blocks the Qi, and the blocked, disturbed Qi keeps the body in a state of unconscious tension while the body loses its ability to achieve a balance by yawning and sleeping, and the lack of sleep blocks the Qi, and so on.

Qigong exercises can break this course of events by means of conscious relaxation of the body.

◆ Is it dangerous if I experience strange sensations when exercising?

Sensations can arise because you may be in a deep meditative condition when exercising. Because such sensations are unfamiliar, they can be disturbing, although they are harmless. To avoid disturbance, keep your attention on the exercise, e.g. observe your body and breathing, take note of the process, and do not be diverted.

This also applies to joyful or pleasant sensations. They are likewise an effect of the exercise. If you begin to concentrate on the sensations rather than the exercise, you are no longer doing Qigong, and its effect, the pleasant experience, will disappear.

In general, pay attention neither to joy nor to anxiety, but let everything come and go and keep your mind on the exercise. If you proceed according to proper instructional standards, no dangerous circumstances can arise.

This is valid for all exercises described in this book. Anyone who practices in accord with another book or instructor, should unconditionally follow their instructions. In any case, if you have little experience in Qigong, you should not attempt to experiment, especially if you have just begun to experience sensations. One who has just begun to ride a bicycle is especially at risk, and one who wants to learn to fly, must first be able to land.

◆ Can I do exercises one after another from different schools?

Take great care if you are practicing exercises with different teachers of Qigong, *Taiji,* Yoga, or Autogenous Training at the same time.

Since exercises of different schools or methods may influence Qi in different ways, different exercises, even different Qigong exercises, can counteract each other. Thus, further Qi-disharmony can result.

It is good, of course, to learn many different kinds of exercises in order to collect experiences. You should, however, follow through on daily practice only with compatible exercises, and in the proper sequence. For the selection and sequence, follow the advice of a Qigong teacher, or an experienced practitioner.

CHAPTER 5

Qigong
For the Advanced

◆ The Healing Tones

In reacting to different circumstances, we produce different sounds. Laughing sounds different than crying. The tone of weeping heals grief's pain, and if you have wept you feel relieved. Tones have influence on your feelings as well as on your body. If you are burdened, you may sigh or groan, and this sound serves to dissipate physical or mental tension. The body demands such a tone and method of breathing to relieve itself.

You should not suppress laughing or crying because the body needs both. Nature does not allow you to laugh if you must cry, and to cry if you must laugh.

By observation and experience of the body, it was discovered that many infirmities can be alleviated or cured by specific sounds. They can be sounds which remain the same, or change, and they can vary in volume and pitch. These sounds consist of vowels and combinations of vowels. Several Qigong exercises have been developed that produce sounds to influence the Qi, the mind, and certain parts of the body. These exercises are done mostly when standing, some when sitting, with or without movement, and with different breathing techniques.

The pitch and variation of the tone, together with the relevant breathing techniques, shape of the mouth, and position and movement of the body, produces an impulse that directly influences the Qi in certain parts of the body. Different tones produce different qualities of impulses in the body. If the body is relaxed, this will cause the Qi to flow. Some exercises are performed in silence with only the mouth forming the shape of the sound.

In Chinese the healing tones are represented by characters; if they are transcribed, an American or European can easily pronounce them. These are natural sounds, appropriate for everyone, and there is no need to "Westernize" them. Weeping or laughing in the West is the same as in China and the rest of the world. Since these sounds are based on natural reactions, it makes no sense to classify them as Chinese, and to want to reform them for use in the rest of the world.

You should note that the same sound is often represented in different Chinese characters which are pronounced very differently in official Chinese (Mandarin). Ancient authors probably spoke different dialects, and therefore gave to the same sound different characters, or used the same character for different sounds. To exercise correctly and produce the correct sound, it is not enough to have only the Chinese character, but also necessary to take into account its origin and pronunciation.

◆ Introduction to the Theory of the Five Phases of Transformation (or Elements)

The doctrine of the five phases of transformation (sometimes also translated as The Doctrine of the Five Elements) is an important component of Chinese philosophy and medicine. The mutual effect of the five elements is the main subject of consideration.

The five elements (*Wu Cai*) are: wood, fire, earth, metal and water. In Chinese history they are regarded as the most important basic elements. In *Shang Shu* it is written: "water and fire are necessary for cooking, metal and wood for working, and earth for growth." By means of observation and reflection this idea developed into the theory of the five elements and their transformations, and summarized and explained the world principle. They have become abstract symbols, and thus no longer represent the elements as such, but five properties or qualities (see the table on the equivalences of the five phases of transformation (elements), p. 110).

They have two sorts of relationship with one another, which are designated as five phases of transformation (*Wu Xing*).

1) Each element produces another, and is, in turn, produced by another. Wood becomes fire, fire becomes earth, earth becomes metal, metal becomes water, and water becomes wood.

It is understood as follows: If wood is burned, these is fire. When the fire dies down, there are ashes which become earth; or by means of fire, earth appears; from earth is produced metal; with metal formed into a tool, you can find water in the ground, and the water brought to the earth's surface allows plants, trees, and thus wood, to grow.

2) Each element overcomes another, and is overcome by another. Water overcomes fire, fire overcomes metal, metal overcomes wood, wood overcomes earth, and

earth overcomes water. You can understand it as follows: water extinguishes fire, fire melts metal, metal chops wood, wood overgrows the earth, and earth can dam up water.

These two enclosed cycles stand again in reciprocal dependence:

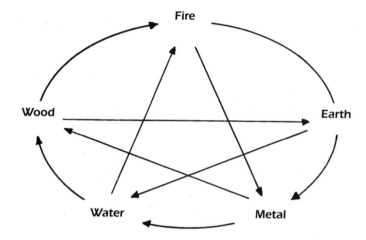

The entire cycle of elements is always affected, never only a part of it. Disharmony in a single area affects the whole system. Thus when converting the theory into diagnosis and therapy, you must look at the system as a whole.

If too little fire prevails, that is not only because there is too little wood, but also because water is present or too much earth consumed, and fire, as mother of earth, suffers. Too much water can indicate the presence of too much metal or too little earth. In this way the reciprocal relations of the organic systems are also represented. The interrelated circles of the five elements, that is, the five phases of transformation, explain the basic functions of the organism. This is determined by observation and experience of the body, and only in regard to these are the elements important for Chinese medicine.

Table of the correspondences of the five transformation phases (elements) in the Macro- and Microcosm.

		Wood	Fire	Earth	Metal	Water
Five Tones	*Wuyin*	Jue (Guo)	Zhi	Gong	Shang	Yu
Five Tastes	*Wuwei*	Sour	Bitter	Sweet	Sharp	Salty
Five Basic Colors	*Wuse*	Blue (Green)	Red	Yellow	White	Black
Five Changes	*Wuhua*	Sprouting, Springing up	Growing	Changing	Harvesting	Storing
Five Climates	*Wuqi*	Wind	Heat	Moisture	Dryness	Cold
Five Directions	*Wufang*	East	South	Center	West	North
Five Seasons	*Wuji*	Spring	Summer	Late Summer (Sixth Chinese Month)	Fall	Winter
Five Transformation Phases (Element)	*Wuxing*	Wood	Fire	Earth	Metal	Water
Zang Organs	*Wuzang*	Liver	Heart	Spleen	Lungs	Kidneys
Fu Organs	*Liufu*	Gall	Small Intestine	Stomach	Large Intestine	Bladder
Five Openings of the Body	*Wuqiao*	Eyes	Tongue, Ears	Mouth	Nose	Ears, Anus, External Genitalia
Five Essential Materials of the Body	*Xingti*	Muscle, Tendon	Arteries and Veins	Flesh	Skin, Hair	Bones
Five Emotions	*Qingzhi*	Anger, Rage	Delight, Joy	Deliberation, Brooding	Sadness, Grief	Fear, Anxiety
Five Sounds	*Wusheng*	Shouting, Screaming	Laughing	Singing	Crying	Groaning
Five Reactions	*Biandong*	Grasping, Making a Fist	Being Worried	Hiccuping	Coughing	Trembling

110

◆ Introduction to the Meridian System

The meridian system consists of different Qi channels *(Mai)*.
They are subdivided into:

- elongated, extended main lines, the meridians *(Jing)*.
- smaller branches formed like a net *(Luo)*
- even smaller branches *(Sun)*

There are twelve meridians, which bear the names of the organ system to which they lead. If for example the "lung" is spoken of, it often means not only the organ in the anatomical sense, but also the Lung Meridian, and everything that it influences (see the table on the correspondences of the five elements in the macrocosm - and microcosm, p. 110). They are divided into four groups:

The three Yin-Meridians of the hand (flow to the hands) are:

- Lung-Meridian *(Fei Jing)*
- Pericardial-Meridian *(Xin Bao Jing)*
- Heart-Meridian *(Xin Jing)*

The three Yang-Meridians of the hand (flow from the hands) are:

- Colon-Meridian *(Da Chang Jing)*
- Triple Burner-Meridian *(San Jiao Jing)*
- Small Intestine-Meridian *(Xiao Chang Jing)*

The three Yang-Meridians of the foot (flow to the feet) are:

- Stomach-Meridian *(Wei Jing)*
- Gallbladder-Meridian *(Dan Jing)*
- Urinary bladder-Meridian *(Pang Guang Jing)*

The three Yin-Meridians of the foot (flow from the feet) are:

- Spleen-Meridian *(Pi Jing)*
- Liver-Meridian *(Gan Jing)*
- Kidney-Meridian *(Shen Jing)*

The meridians have definite directions of flow. Generally, the three Yin-Meridians of the hand lead from the chest along the inside of the arms to the hand. There they connect with the three Yang-Meridians of the hands, travel through the back of the hands and along the outsides of the arms to the head and face. There they connect to the three

Yang-Meridians of the feet, which lead from the head and face mainly through the front, back and sides of the body to the feet. From there the three Yin-Meridians of the feet lead mainly from the inner sides of the legs through the lower abdomen to the chest. Here they connect with the three Yin-Meridians of the hands and the circuit is closed.

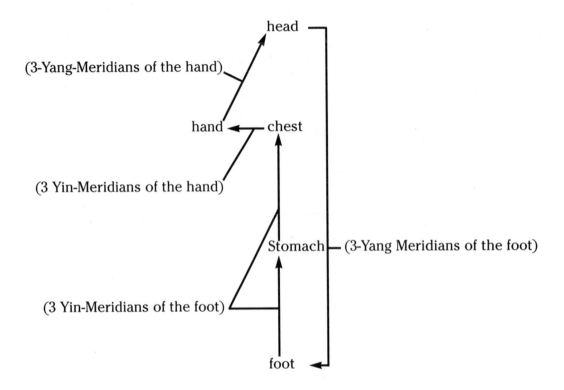

The exact circuit is displayed in the following illustrations:

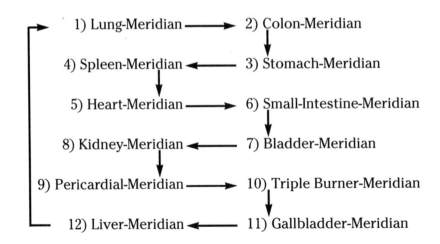

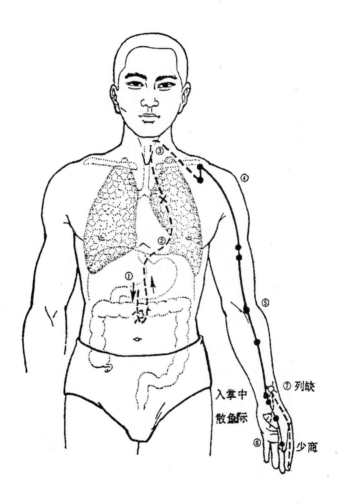

入掌中
散魚際

⑦ 列缺

⑥ 少商

Lung-Meridian (Fei Jing)

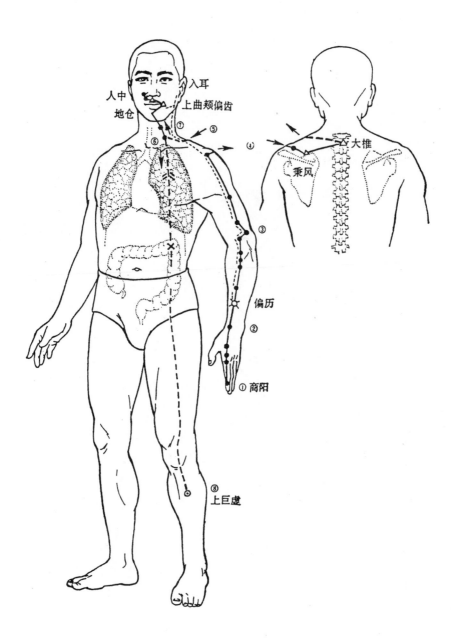

入耳
人中
上曲頰偏齒
地仓
⑦
⑤
④
⑥
大椎
秉风
③
偏历
②
① 商阳
⑧ 上巨虚

Colon-(large-intestine) Meridian (Da Chang Jing)

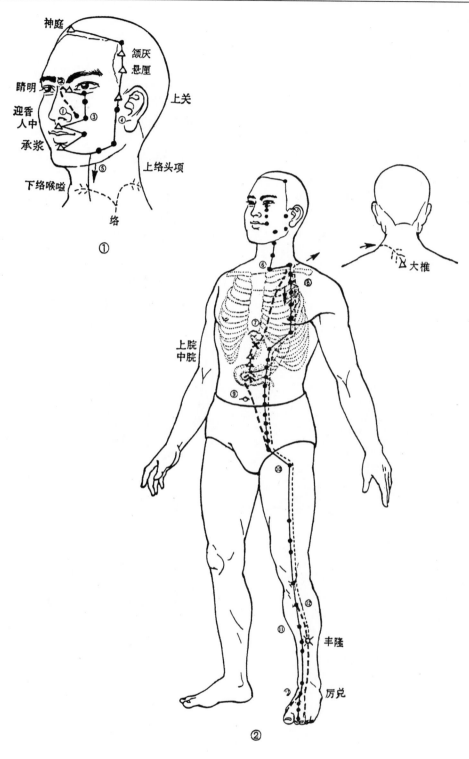

神庭
颔厌
悬厘
上关
睛明
迎香
人中
承浆
上络头项
下络喉咙
络
①

大椎

上脘
中脘

丰隆

厉兑

②

Stomach-Meridian (Wei Jing)

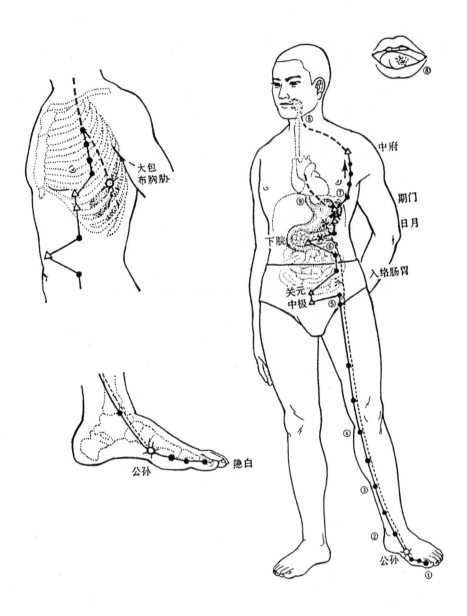

中府
期门
日月
入络肠胃
关元
中极
下脘
大包
布胸胁
公孙
隐白
公孙

Spleen-Meridian (Pi Jing)

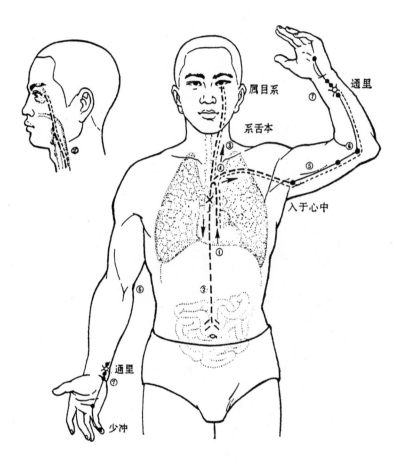

属目系

系舌本

入于心中

通里

少冲

通里

Heart-Meridian (Xin Jing)

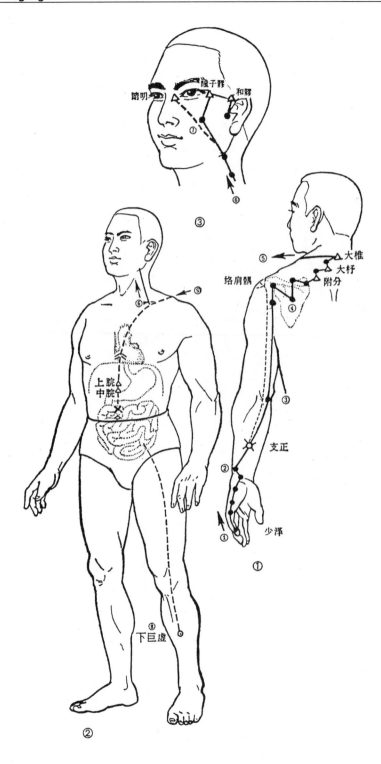

Small Intestine-Meridian (Xiao Chang Jing)

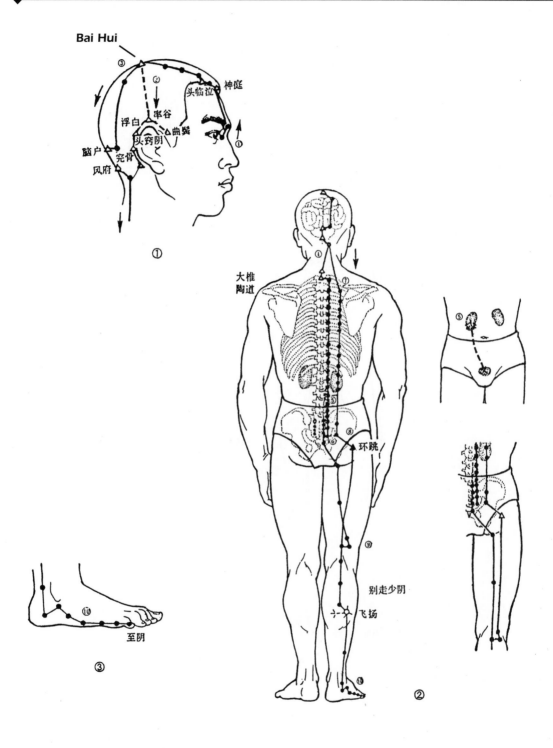

Bai Hui

Bai Hui

③

④

头临泣

神庭

率谷

浮白

曲鬓

头窍阴

脑户

完骨

风府

①

大椎

陶道

④

⑦

⑤

⑧

环跳

别走少阴

飞扬

⑨

⑩

至阴

③

②

Bladder-Meridian (Pang Guang Jing)

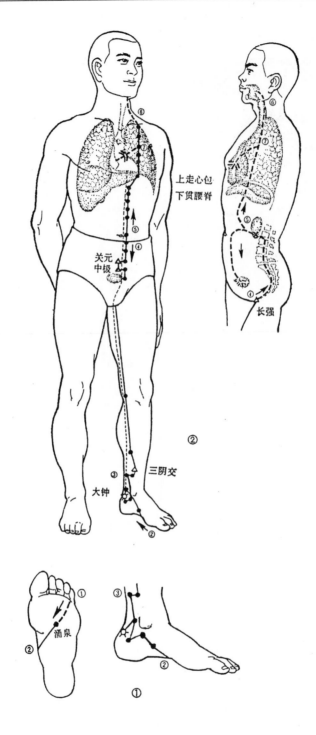

上走心包
下贯腰脊

关元
中极

长强

三阴交

大钟

涌泉

Kidney-Meridian (Shen Jing)

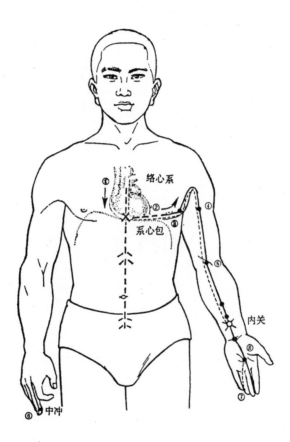

Pericardial-Meridian (Xin Bao Jing)

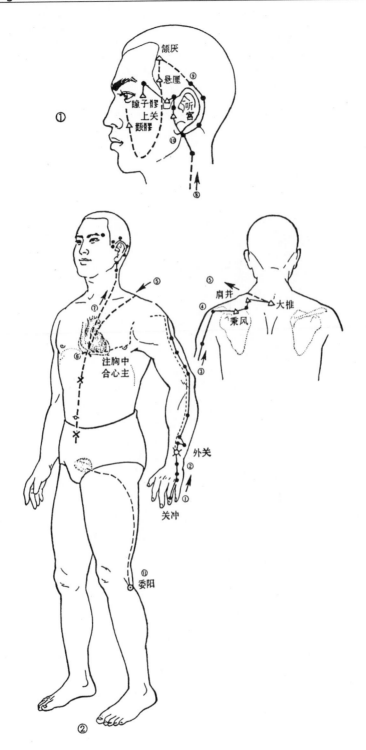

Triple Burner-Meridian (San Jiao Jing)

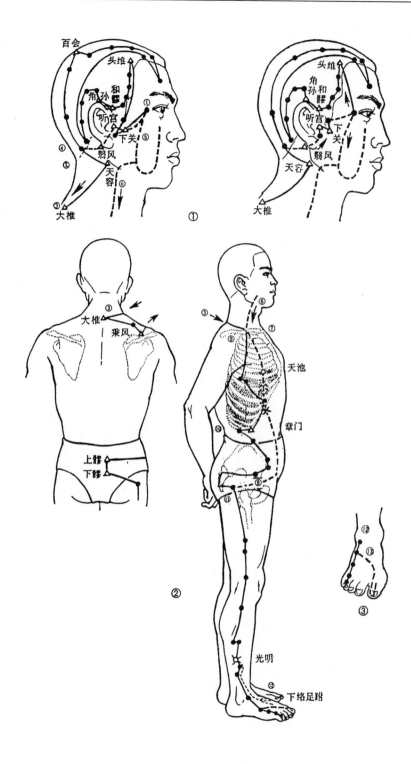

Gallbladder-Meridian (Dan Jing)

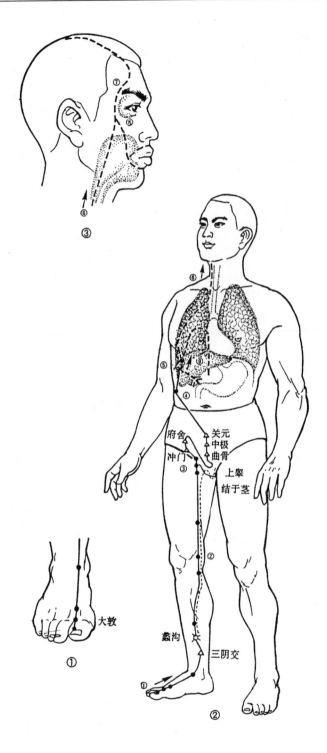

Liver-Meridian (Gan Jing)

There are also Meridians which do not lead directly to an inner organ. They form connections between the Meridians, and are named according to their functions. They are the so-called "irregular" Meridians *(Qi Jing Ba Mai or Ji Jing Ba Mai).*

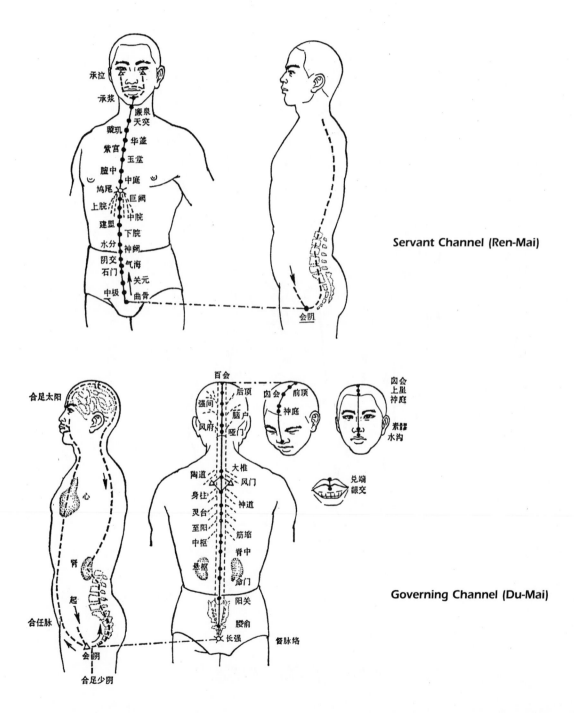

Servant Channel (Ren-Mai)

Governing Channel (Du-Mai)

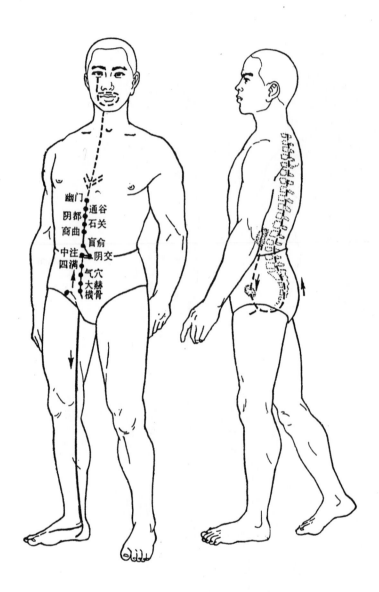

幽门
阴都
商曲
中注
四满

通谷
石关
肓俞
阴交
气穴
大赫
横骨

Nodal Point Channel (Chong Mai)

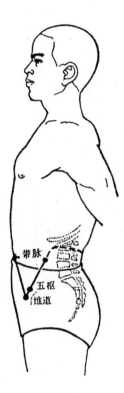

带脉

五枢
维道

Girdle Vessel (Dai-Mai)

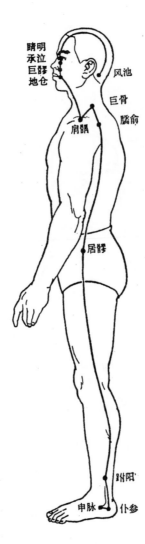

睛明
承泣
巨髎
地仓

风池

巨骨
臑俞

肩髃

居髎

跗阳

申脉 仆参

Heel-Yang Channel (Yang Qiao-Mai)

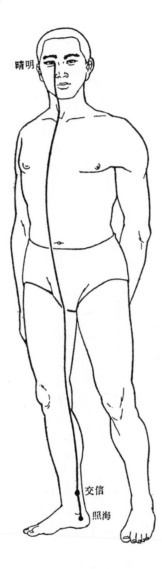

晴明

交信
照海

Heel-Yin Channel (Yin-Qiao-Mai)

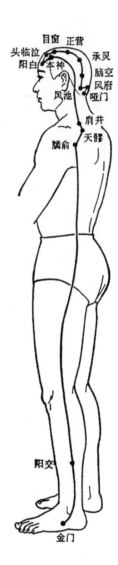

目窗　正营
头临泣
阳白
本神
承灵
脑空
风府
风池
哑门
肩井
天髎
臑俞
阳交
金门

Yang-Connecting Channel (Yang-Wei-Mai)

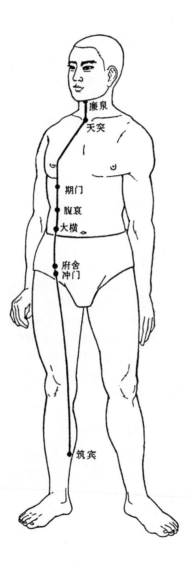

廉泉

天突

期门

腹哀

大横

府舍
冲门

筑宾

Yin-Connecting Channel (Yin-Wei-Mai)

◆ Function of the Meridians

1) Produces connections between:

- the jointly functioning organ pair *Zang* (corresponds to Yin) and *Fu* (corresponds to Yang) which are a pair designated as through one of the five elements. *Zang* can be translated as store-house, and *Fu* as renovator, palace, or residence (see the Table on the correspondences of the five elements and the chapter on Yin-Yang, p.110);

- inner organs, and body openings or sense organs: eyes, ears, nose, mouth, tongue, external sex organs, and anus;

- inner organs and the periphery, for example, between the lungs and the thumb tip.

2) Transportation of Qi

The Qi can flow through the Meridians. Good and bad influences are directed in the same way through the channels.

3) Reflection of the inner organs

You can observe, on a road leading to a city, if it is raining in the city because outward bound cars will be wet. You can also, by means of the Meridians, know whether the inner organs are in order. Since all inner organs have a Meridian which leads to the periphery of the body, signs of disturbances and illnesses of the inner organs can always be found at corresponding positions in the Meridians. In Traditional Chinese Medicine wholly independent diagnostic methods have been developed on this principle, which are completely different from Western diagnostic methods.

4. Regulation of Xu (empty) and Shi (full)

If a Qi disharmony occurs in the body, it can be treated by acting on the Meridians. Through application of acupuncture needles at specific places on the Meridians, the Qi there, when there is too little or none at all *(Xü)*, can be replenished; and when there is too much *(Shi)*, it can be lead away. Through the Meridians all organ systems can be harmonized with the Qi (in the sense of Yin and Yang), so that the body is balanced and united.

To quote an important sentence about the Meridians from one Qigong classic *Huang Di Nei Jing: "The Meridians determine life and death, treat all illnesses, regulate Xü and Shi, and ought not to be blocked."*

◆ Yin and Yang

Yin and Yang originally meant shadows and sun, or the dark and light side of a thing. They express no judgment, but only characterize all opposites; for example, inside and outside, below and above, right and left, night and day, women and men, winter and summer.

The Yin-Yang principle only has a meaning when both parts of opposite pairs are compared. Nothing in and of itself can be characterized as Yin or Yang. Summer can only be characterized as Yang if it is considered as the opposite to winter. Both parts of a contrasting pair must also be comparable. For example, it is not possible to contrast summer as Yang with night as Yin since they are not opposite to one another.

Yang is also contained in Yin and vice versa. Summer (Yang) consists of days (Yang) and nights (Yin). Yin and Yang can change into one another as summer passes away, and fall and winter approach.

The Yin-Yang principle is a law of nature with which Chinese philosophy and TCM explain the microcosm and macrocosm and how they change.

The Qi-Harmonizer: OMNI-MOBIL

Our modern society suffers increasingly from lack of movement. Millions of people have back pains and joint problems. According to Traditional Chinese Medicine (TMC) theses pains are caused by a blockage of Qi, the life energy, in parts of the back and joints. The acupuncture-analgesic of TMC, which has been recommended by the World Health Organization (WHO), proves the fact that no pain can exist wherever this energy is harmonized within the body. TCM is based on the principle that "Qi-harmony is health itself." Following this principle, Chinese physician and Qigong master Qingshan Liu has developed the first Qi-Harmonizer, the OMNI-MOBIL.

With the OMNI-MOBIL you can directly achieve Qi-harmony, which can't be done with the usual fitness equipment. Most equipment trains only single muscles in isolation. Even the so-called 'total-body-trainers' such rowers and ski-machines only exercise the muscles of certain body parts through one-sided strain. This kind of training builds up your muscles, but strong muscles don't necessarily mean that you are healthy and well-balanced.

On the other hand, the Qi-Harmonizer provides a varied and balanced exertion of the whole body through a smooth, flowing sequence of movements. The exercise movements consist of special combinations of stretching, bending, pulling, and expanding, just like in many Qigong exercises. In addition, the equipment itself offers resistance in both directions. This activates the Yang-Meridians (e.g. the flexor muscles of the arms) as well as the Yin-Meridians (e.g. the extensor muscles of the arms), just like the Qi flows in its natural course from the Yin-Meridian to the Yang-Meridian. This flow of energy dissolves Qi-blockages and can eliminate the causes of a variety of tensions, pains, and diseases. Moreover, this kind of training requires little exertion while making you feel good and keeping you healthy. The OMNI-MOBIL is therefore the first high-tech exercise equipment developed according to the ancient and well-proven principles of Traditional Chinese Medicine. It may be produced as a stationary machine or even as a bicycle.

The OMNI-MOBIL has been awarded first prize in the field of health and fitness at the largest international inventor's fairs; INPEX IX (USA), IENA, and EUREKA (Europe). Many international television stations such as CNN, ARD, and ZDF, as well as prestigious newspapers and magazines, have reported on this invention.

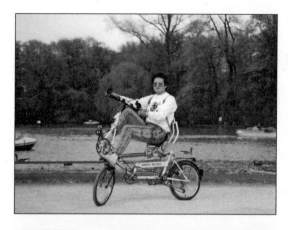
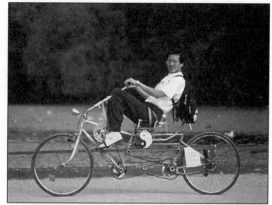
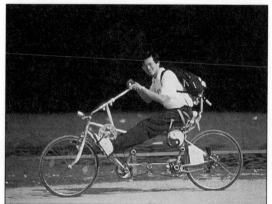
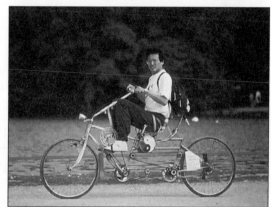

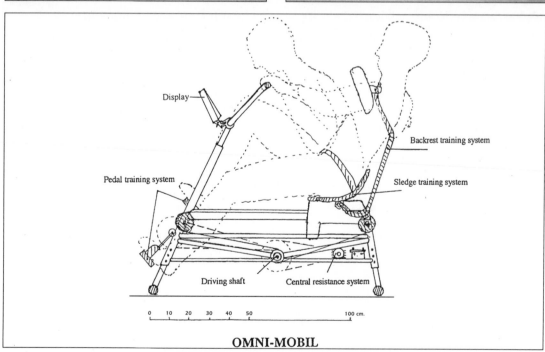

Display

Backrest training system

Pedal training system

Sledge training system

Driving shaft

Central resistance system

0 10 20 30 40 50   100 cm.

OMNI-MOBIL

Seminars with Qingshan Liu

Getting healthy and staying healthy
for yourself and for others

- Experience the thousands of years old secret techniques of **Authentic Medical Qigong (AMQ)**
- Training course to become a certified Qigong teacher for integration into therapeutic professions and use in the health care services.

Qingshan Liu, Qigong master and Chinese doctor, has completed the training of his students as Qigong teachers within 14 months of intensive instruction and after a rigorous exam on January 14, 1996. During this training they had, as the first Europeans ever, the opportunity to become familiar with exercise techniques that for thousands of years had remained secret and had been passed on to only a few chosen disciples.

Using those techniques enabled them to learn new exercises much faster, look at exercises they already knew from a completely new perspective and enter different realms of experience with a heightened intensity. They used more direct ways and achieved the goal of the exercises faster. This is why some students could become excellent Qigong teachers within such a short time. During this comprehensive training course they learned a variety of exercises which are still unknown in Europe. The training has been officially acknowledged by several health insurance companies.

This special training program excels because of its well-aimed systematic approach to the final objective of the course: the "grasping" of the essence of Qigong by perceiving the positive effects of the exercises. Those have been carefully selected so that they support each other and harmonize together. Furthermore, special attention is given to the therapeutic effects of particular exercises on certain diseases. Inner visualizations of the Meridian system and the practice of perceiving and directing the Qi will make you realize and understand the essence of Traditional Chinese Medicine (TMC). Now you know the meaning of Qigong and you can continue learning and teaching on your own.

Important: The training program also serves as a Qigong cure. Only after you have experienced the healing effects of the exercises on your own body and soul and acquired a complete command of the exercise techniques are you able to really help other people —competently, with love, and with all your heart.

◆ The Training Program

PART I: *(150 lessons)*

Section 1: *Harmony in body and soul; fit and vital for the daily routine:*
Qigong harmony in 18 figures and 8 exercises for daily life:

You begin with the basics of Qigong practice and experience a very soft, balancing series of exercises with a harmonious sequence of 18 figures and 8 exercises for daily life. These are easy to learn, can be practiced separately, and have a positive effect on many widespread ailments. Furthermore they are a good preparation for learning AMQ and Taijiquan.

Section 2: *Systematic Instruction in AMQ*

You begin with the basics of AMQ practice and learn during the training a variety of traditional exercises (standing, sitting, lying, and walking). The selected still and moving exercise techniques and healing sounds are combined in an organic and very meaningful way. The special combination leads to a fast increase and deepening of your knowledge of Qigong in general and enables you to perform the important AMQ-exercises correctly. There are 8 topics:

- Strengthening of the immune system; solves back and joint problems
- Strengthening of the kidney system; solves insomnia and bone problems
- Improvement of memory and concentration; heart and circulation
- Regulation of the cooperation of all organ systems
- Strengthening of the lung system; becoming one with the cosmos
- Regulation of digestion; stabilizes inner balance and serenity
- Yin-Yang-Harmonizing with the Qigong stick
- Healthy vitality and sexuality; joy of living

PART II: *(180 lessons)*

Practical and Theoretical Teacher's Training

- Recognizing and understanding the background and the meaning of exercise movements and techniques by systematic analysis and comparison of previously-learned exercises and elements of exercises.
- Capability to detect faults in other's exercises, to correct the exercises and explain their effects (which under certain circumstances can be detrimental).
- By perceiving the Qi you will sense the Meridian system and by AMQ you will get to know and experience the principles of Traditional Chinese Medicine (TMC).

There is no need to learn the principles of TMC by heart, but by "touching," experiencing and perceiving you will reach the inexhaustible source of TMC and move along with self-confidence in the rivers of cognition.

- Learning to combine specific suitable exercises as therapy against certain diseases
- Didactic of teaching, supervision and group dynamics
- Introduction and eventual practical use of the Chinese science of nutrition
- Introduction into Tuina-Anmo healing massage
- Introduction into Chinese health care. Wisdom from the *Classic of the Yellow Emperor,* the oldest literature of TMC.

This part of the program lasts 4 weeks in total. Each week, however, is separate with intervals of 3 to 4 months in between so that students have sufficient time to practice at home.

You may contact the author about these programs at:

Qingshan Liu
P.O. Box 81 05 41
D-81905 Munich
Germany

Tel: 011-49-89-9295663
Fax: 011-49-89-9296752

A P P E N D I X   C

Qigong Retreat

◆ Qigong in Majorca

- Draw energy from plants and nature
- Life energy and serenity through Qigong exercises with plants
- A Chinese secret thousands of years old known among only a few monks in China
  Now being introduced in the USA by Master Liu in an authentic way

Discover the secret in a Mediterranean climate under the optimal conditions of the plant world. Experience these unique Qigong vacations with us in Majorca.

In a very special, carefully selected site in Majorca with a suitable plant world we begin the early morning exercises at sunrise in order to get to know the Qi of nature and plants, which is at that time of the day especially active, and let it have its positive effect on us. We learn to perceive the Qi of different plants and to gather it through still and moving exercise techniques (about 2 hours).

The rest of the day is at your disposal for excursions, sightseeing, leisure time activities or exercises on your own. If you wish, you also have the opportunity of individual consultation with Master Liu.

In the evening there is time for answering questions, discussions of any problems that might have occurred during the exercises, and exchange of experience. Furthermore, we perform exercises which help us perceive the Qi of the night hours.

On one of the first mornings beginners have the option to participate in a general introduction to Qigong. In an additional seminar (approximately 2 hours) you will get acquainted with practical elements of Tuina-Anmo therapeutic massage, a technique which promises a healing effect especially on back and joint problems as well as tensions and exhaustion. You will also get an introduction to the basic principles of Traditional Chinese Medicine, the Meridian system and special acupuncture points. The course is rounded off by an authentic introduction to Taijiquan.

Location: Our four-star hotel is situated in the middle of a 23,000 square meter park-like pine forest, away from crowded tourist areas, 24 kilometers south-east from Palma. This area provides optimal conditions for the exercises. The beach is approximately 800 meters from the hotel, which offers a wide variety of leisure-time activities.

Duration: One week (for detailed information please contact the address on the previous page).

◆ Weight Regulation and Agility with Qigong

- Wellness of body and soul
- Vitality and joy of living
- Harmonizing of body movements
- Healthy nutrition

"The usual negative side effects of weight control methods known in Western societies are completely absent here. You won't feel cold or frustrated, nor hungry or tired! On the contrary: you will experience a lot of power and stamina, good sleep, a keen mind and joy of living, an increasing agility and enormous loss of weight (5 kg during the first week)."

(Quotation of a seminar student)

You too can experience activating the self-regulating forces of the body with Master Liu's exercises. Let your body find its ideal weight without going hungry or fasting—no matter if you are too slim or too heavy. These special inner visualizations, breathing techniques and harmonious movements are easy to learn and will make you generally more well-balanced, fit and efficient. You will feel more power and joy of living! With Master Liu you can test these Qigong techniques, proven for thousands of years.

Dates: 2 days, e.g. Weekend, 10:00 A.M. until 5:00 P.M.

You may contact the author about these programs at:

Qingshan Liu
P.O. Box 81 05 41
D-81905 Munich
Germany

Tel: 011-49-89-9295663
Fax: 011-49-89-9296752

About the Author

Following his family's tradition, Qingshan Liu has practiced Qigong and *Taijiquan* since childhood. He learned this thousand year old art from famous masters in China and was acknowledged as master even as a youth after he had successfully passed rigorous exams.

Liu studied modern Western Medicine and Traditional Chinese Medicine, including acupuncture, acupressure and *Tuina-Anmo* therapeutic massage in Beijing. Since 1986 he has been teaching Qigong in Germany. His goal is to preserve the quality and authenticity of Qigong in order to help people competently. The Qigong teachers trained by him (some among them are also doctors) have been acknowledged by several health insurance companies.

Qingshan Liu speaks fluent English and German. He is known as book author and by his performances on television (ARD, ZDF) as Qigong master, as well as for the Qigong training equipment "OMNI-MOBIL" which he developed.

Bibliography

Bao Pu Zi by Ge Hong, also known as Bao Pu Zi, of the Eastern Jin dynasty (317–420 A.D.).

Huang Di Nei Jing, shortened to *Nei Jing* (usually translated as *Classic of the Yellow Emperor*), is the oldest classic on Traditional Chinese Medicine. It originates from about the time of the warring empires (475–221 B.C.).

Nan Jing, originates from about the Western Han period (206 B.C.–24 A.D.). Its alleged author Bian Que lived, however, at the time of the warring empires (475–221 B.C.) and is a very famous figure in Chinese medicine.

Qigong de Ke Xue Ji Chu by Xie Huan Zhang, Peking TU Press, 1988.

Shang Shu, a historic book on the prehistoric period. According to legend, Confucius is the author.

Tai Qing Tiao Qi Jing. The author is unknown, but the book is presumed to be from the Tang dynasty (618–907 A.D.), and is a classic Qigong book.

Wu Yao Yuan Quan by Wang Ang of the Qing dynasty (1644–1912 A.D.), is one of the most important works on Qigong.

Yi, an abbreviation for *Zhou Yi*, consists of two main parts *Yi Jing (I Ching)* and *Yi Zhuan*. It is one of the oldest and most important collections of Confucian texts and dates approximately from the 2100 to 476 B.C.

Zhuang Zi Zhi Bei Jou, comes from the time of the warring empires (475–221 B.C.).

Index

Books & Videos from YMAA

YMAA Publication Center Books

B005. *CHI KUNG — Health and Martial Arts*
B006. *NORTHERN SHAOLIN SWORD*
B007R. *TAI CHI THEORY & MARTIAL POWER — Advanced Yang Style Tai Chi Chuan (formerly Adv. Yang Style Tai Chi v.1)*
B008R. *TAI CHI CHUAN MARTIAL APPLICATIONS — Advanced Yang Style Tai Chi Chuan (formerly Adv. Yang Style Tai Chi v.2)*
B009. *ANALYSIS OF SHAOLIN CHIN NA — Instructor's Manual*
B010R. *EIGHT SIMPLE QIGONG EXERCISES FOR HEALTH*
B011R. *THE ROOT OF CHINESE QIGONG — The Secrets of Chi Kung Training*
B012. *MUSCLE/TENDON CHANGING AND MARROW/BRAIN WASHING CHI KUNG — The Secret of Youth*
B013. *HSING YI CHUAN — Theory and Applications*
B014. *THE ESSENCE OF TAI CHI CHI KUNG — Health and Martial Arts*
B015R. *ARTHRITIS — The Chinese Way of Healing and Prevention (formerly Qigong for Arthritis)*
B016. *CHINESE QIGONG MASSAGE — General Massage*
B017R. *HOW TO DEFEND YOURSELF — Effective & Practical Martial Arts Strategies*
B018. *THE TAO OF BIOENERGETICS — East – West*
B019R. *SIMPLIFIED TAI CHI CHUAN — 24 & 48 Postures with Martial Applications (formerly A Guide to Taijiquan)*
B020. *BAGUAZHANG — Emei Baguazhang*
B021. *COMPREHENSIVE APPLICATIONS OF SHAOLIN CHIN NA — The Practical Defense of Chinese Seizing Arts for All Styles*
B022. *TAIJI CHIN NA — The Seizing Art of Taijiquan*
B023. *PROFESSIONAL BUDO — Ethics, Chivalry, and the Samurai Code*
B024. *SONG OF A WATER DRAGON — Biography of He Yi An*
B025. *THE ESSENCE OF SHAOLIN WHITE CRANE — Martial Power and Qigong*
B026. *OPENINGS — A Zen Joke Guide for Serious Problem Solving*
B027. *WISDOM'S WAY — 101 Tales of Chinese Wit*
B028. *CHINESE FAST WRESTLING — The Art of San Shou Kuai Jiao*
B029. *CHINESE FITNESS — A Mind/Body Approach*
B030. *BACK PAIN — Chinese Qigong for Healing and Prevention*

YMAA Publication Center Children's Books

CB001. *CARVING THE BUDDHA*
CB002. *THE MASK OF THE KING*
CB003. *THE FOX BORROWS THE TIGER'S AWE*

YMAA Publication Center Videotapes

T001. *YANG STYLE TAI CHI CHUAN — and Its Applications*
T002. *SHAOLIN LONG FIST KUNG FU — Lien Bu Chuan and Its Applications*
T003. *SHAOLIN LONG FIST KUNG FU — Gung Li Chuan and Its Applications*
T004. *SHAOLIN CHIN NA*
T005. *THE EIGHT PIECES OF BROCADE — Wai Dan Chi Kung Exercise Set*
T006. *CHI KUNG FOR TAI CHI CHUAN*
T007. *QIGONG FOR ARTHRITIS — The Chinese Way of Healing and Prevention*
T008. *CHINESE QIGONG MASSAGE — Self Massage*
T009. *CHINESE QIGONG MASSAGE — Massage with a Partner*
T010. *HOW TO DEFEND YOURSELF 1 — Unarmed Attack*
T011. *HOW TO DEFEND YOURSELF 2 — Knife Attack*
T012. *COMPREHENSIVE APPLICATIONS OF SHAOLIN CHIN NA 1*
T013. *COMPREHENSIVE APPLICATIONS OF SHAOLIN CHIN NA 2*
T014. *SHAOLIN LONG FIST KUNG FU — Yi Lu Mai Fu & Er Lu Mai Fu and their Applications*
T015. *SHAOLIN LONG FIST KUNG FU — Shi Zi Tang and its Applications*
T016. *TAIJI CHIN NA*
T017. *EMEI BAGUAZHANG 1 — Basic Training, Qigong, Eight Palms, & their Applications*
T018. *EMEI BAGUAZHANG 2 — Swimming Body & its Applications*
T019. *EMEI BAGUAZHANG 3 — Bagua Deer Hook Swords & its Applications*
T020. *XINGYIQUAN — The Twelve Animal Patterns & their Applications*
T021. *TAIJIQUAN — Simplified 24 & 48 Form Sequence (Sequence Only)*
T022. *WU STYLE TAIJIQUAN — with Applications*
T023. *SUN STYLE TAIJIQUAN — with Applications*
T024. *TAIJIQUAN — Simplified 24 Forms with Applications & Simplified 48 Forms*

YMAA Publication Center 楊氏武藝協會

38 Hyde Park Avenue • Jamaica Plain, MA 02130
1-800-669-8892 • email: ymaa@aol.com